THE FAMILY PREGNANCY

THE FAMILY PREGNANCY

A Revolutionary Holistic and Medical Guide to Maternity

MARY JANE BOVO, M.D.

Foreword by Louis Weinstein, M.D.
Illustrations by Michele Donnelly
Photography by Linda Mahon
Research/Indexing by Christine O'Brien

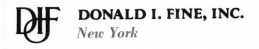

DONALD I. FINE, INC.
New York

Library of Congress Catalogue Card Number: 94-071115

ISBN: 1-55611-418-4

Manufactured in the United States of America

10   9   8   7   6   5   4   3   2   1

Designed by Irving Perkins Associates

FOR SAMUEL

ACKNOWLEDGMENTS

❧ NO PROJECT IS THE WORK OF ONE PERSON. WITH-
out the help, devotion, praise, criticism and encouragement of
many people, this book would never have been a reality.

A very special thank you to Christine O'Brien, for her extraordinary research and impeccable editing, for the emotional support she unfailingly gives me, no matter what the endeavor, for
being the mother of my incredible grandson and for being my
wonderful daughter; to Samuel, my grandson, whose gestation in-
spired this book and who believes his Nini can do anything; and
to Michael O'Brien, my son-in-law, who understood why his wife
stayed up until 4:00 A.M. every morning doing research. A special
thank you to Michele Donnelly, my sister, whose beautiful illustrations clarify what is happening to you and your baby; to Linda
Mahon, whose extraordinary photographs depict what a family
pregnancy really looks like; to Dr. Louis Weinstein, who kept say-
ing, "Write the book, write the book"; to Carol Trenary, my office
manager and personal assistant, who took care of details at the office and awakened me every morning to see patients after I had
been writing all night; to Christine Tutelian, my nurse, who
shared her twenty years of experience in obstetrics; to Elaine
Phipps, who kept me writing; to Allison Mastin, who kept me one
step ahead; to Dr. Steven Gabbe and Dr. Michael Menutti, who
taught me the art and discipline of obstetrics; to Dr. Celso Ramon
Garcia, who always had time for questions and who shared his ex-
pertise in infertility surgery; to Dr. Anthony Mastrian, who
showed me that you should treat patients as individuals; to Nancy
Coffey, my incredible agent, whose encouragement has been endless; to Donald Fine, my publisher, who believed in what I had to
say; to Anthony Favaro, whose retrieval of my lost research made
this all much easier; and to Joseph Santoli, whose professional assistance made a difficult situation better, thus making my deadlines feasible. Thank you to Sue Ferguson of the National Infor-

mation Center for Children and Youth with Disabilities and Marie of the National Association of Childbearing Centers for sharing their knowledge.

A very special thank you to my patients, who believed in my theories, used them and allowed me to be a part of their personal miracle. A grateful thank you to the moms, dads and babies who allowed me to photograph their pregnancies.

—M. J. BOVO

CONTENTS

FOREWORD

WHAT PLEASURE IT IS TO READ A BOOK THAT treats pregnancy as a normal condition, yet gives to the couple the necessary information to enter this most important portion of their lives properly informed. As a practicing obstetrician/gynecologist, a maternal-fetal medicine specialist and a professor and chairperson of the department of obstetrics and gynecology at a university medical school, the focus of my life has been that of an educator. I have learned that it is uncommon for a physician to actually cure a patient. What we should do is be a source of support and information for our patients in order to assist them in the healing process.

Many pregnant patients do not need a health care provider if proper information is available to help them understand the normal physiologic changes that occur during pregnancy. Pregnancy is not a disease and it does not need a cure. It is a time of creation and love when a woman has experiences that a man will never have. How envious I have been of all my patients and my wife when, after 40 weeks of heaven and hell, a new human life is assisted into this hectic world. We can argue and discuss affirmative action and equal employment opportunities, but in the area of the creation of life, a woman has no equal. This role of giving birth and the years of motherhood to follow are truly gifts from God. The sexes may desire equality but in this way they shall always be separate. I could only stand and watch as my wife breast fed our son for 6 months, a continuation of the nourishment she provided for him in the womb.

Mary Jane Bovo and I have been friends since we met when I was giving one of my many lectures to physicians around the country. Our chance meeting has developed into a friendship and mutual respect that has persisted for many years. Mary Jane first talked about this book six years ago, and I was very supportive of her efforts. We agreed that there was a need for a single reference to which women could go to answer questions about the period prior to conception, the time during pregnancy, the delivery process *and* the postpartum period. *The Family Pregnancy* is just such a volume. Here, Dr. Bovo's explanations are clear, simple and answer so many of the questions that physicians often do not spend the time discussing with their patients. Dr. Bovo's case vignettes are appropriately interspersed to support the concepts she is presenting.

An extremely important portion of the book are the appendices. Anyone who looks at these will appreciate the value of the information listed and the concise manner of presentation. This material is a valuable resource for all the needs of the family regarding the new addition.

Being an educator is more than being a teacher—it is a gift that returns itself many-fold as one progresses in her or his respective field; the ability to learn from patients is an asset that many health care providers lack. Similarly, being a doctor is more than having received a medical degree. And being a physician is more than meeting the requirements of the state licensing authority. Finally, to become a healer the individual must realize that lifelong study is a critical component in this goal. *The Family Pregnancy* demonstrates that Dr. Bovo has reached this goal to the extent that she is willing both to teach and to learn from her patients. You, the reader, have an excellent opportunity to learn and understand the changes that will occur to the mother and to the family during pregnancy. You will learn from *The Family Pregnancy* how to share your experiences with your family and friends. In turn, be sure to teach your doctor about yourself and your needs. You deserve the best, and with the information gleaned from these pages you will be able to grow and share in this most beautiful of life's events.

From one healer to another, well done, Mary Jane.

—LOUIS WEINSTEIN, M.D.
May 18, 1994

PREFACE

PLANNING A PREGNANCY USED TO BE A LUXURY and dependent only on finances. Now it's a necessity for the well-being of mom, dad and baby.

We now know that we can reduce the occurrence of many birth defects through diet, exercise and the use of vitamins before conception. Prenatal conditioning may produce calmer, more responsive babies. In addition, such planning helps the father feel a part of the exciting, sometimes terrifying, process.

Having a child is one of the most important decisions we make in life. It should also be one of the best prepared for events. Many times a woman is four, five or six weeks pregnant before she realizes that she and her partner have started a new life. At this point, major organ systems have already begun to form and the things we do in everyday life may have already caused the baby to have an unhealthy start.

We expect our partners to be supportive during our pregnancies, but have we included them in the planning as well as the doing? Have we considered their health and how it contributes to a healthy baby? Have we thought about how our habits affect our baby, how our pregnancy affects other family members, our co-workers, even our own daily life? Have we chosen where our baby will be delivered and by whom? Have we thought about how this pregnancy will affect both mom and dad's emotions and daily life?

The nineties are a time of quality time to be spent on the things that matter most to us, a time to get in touch with each other and be a family, whatever that family unit may consist of. In my own practice, I consult with families of every imaginable combination. One thing all my couples have in common, however, is a desire to provide the best possible beginning for their child. The concerns of both mom and dad before, during and after pregnancy are addressed, so that we truly have a family pregnancy.

This book is intended to be a guide to achieving that beginning, to furthering the bond and becoming closer while awaiting the birth of your child and to going home as a family unit. It will give you practical suggestions as well as basic medical advice about your preconception time, your pregnancy and delivery and your return home with your permanent houseguest.

CHAPTER ONE

TO BE OR NOT TO BE

Making the Decision
Choosing the Practitioner,
Place and Method

❦ TWELVE MONTHS OF PREGNANCY? ISN'T NINE enough? Family pregnancy? I'm the one who'll be pregnant! These could be your thoughts as you start to read this book. In fact, you could already be pregnant.

A twelve-month pregnancy means planning, getting pregnant, being pregnant and using fetal conditioning, involving your partner in the pregnancy, having the baby and going home as a new family. This book will give you basic medical advice that along with your health care practitioner can help you have a healthy, happy, stress-free pregnancy. It is intended to help you make choices and to show you why planning for your pregnancy and learning to become a new family are some of the most important things you and your partner will do together.

MAKING THE DECISION

Making the decision to start or add to a family is not a simple one. Pregnancy will involve all aspects of your lives: emotional, physical, financial, career and relational.

You and your partner must look at your motivations for wanting to be parents and what it means to each of you. By answering the following questions, you can begin discussions to honestly make this life-altering decision.

1. Are we a stable couple?
2. Will we share responsibilities of child care, home care?

3. Are we the same religion? If not, does this pose a problem for the child's religious training?
4. Will a child add to our relationship?
5. Do we have similar ideas about education, discipline?
6. How will having a baby affect our careers?
7. Can we afford a baby? (See Table 1-1)
8. Can we afford child care?
9. Do we have a support system near us, if needed?
10. Do we have an emotional support system, if needed?
11. If we had to support a parent or sibling (emotionally, financially, physically), could we do this with a child?
12. Will our insurance cover maternity and newborn expenses? (If not, now is the time to change your coverage to include maternity/newborn/well-child expenses.)

You and your partner should honestly discuss these and other issues that may arise before you get pregnant. You should both agree that the time is right for a pregnancy.

TIMING IS EVERYTHING

Lisa, a twenty-eight-year-old patient of mine, came in to see me in an absolute state of elation. She had missed her period and was sure she was pregnant. "I've been married for over three years. My husband and I discussed having children before we got married, so four months ago I decided to stop the pill. I want a baby and I know Jeff will be happy."

I spent over an hour discussing pregnancy and the effect it would have on her life and marriage if she were indeed pregnant. I spoke to Lisa about the couple's finances and was astounded when Lisa informed me that her husband had lost his job as a Wall Street corporate VP. Upon questioning her further, I discovered that Lisa knew exactly when in her cycle she could get pregnant.

"Jeff doesn't know I stopped taking the pill. Why should I have told him? We discussed children before marriage. I want to stop working and start a family, and this feels like the right time for me."

Lisa left the office elated, because I did confirm her pregnancy. She said she was taking Jeff out to dinner to break the news. Two weeks later, Lisa returned for her first prenatal visit. She was obviously upset and said, "Dr. Bovo, Jeff is not happy about this pregnancy. We both want a child so much, but I guess my timing was off." I suggested Jeff come for the next visit, even though he was reluctant to "get involved" with this baby.

During that next visit, I discussed with them the possibility of going to a financial counselor, Jeff's options in the workplace and Lisa's agreement to stay at work a few months longer. Jeff did want the child, but he was frightened and felt deceived.

Jeff and Lisa decided to proceed with the pregnancy and worked to improve the lines of communication between them. This had now become a family pregnancy that could be shared.

Pregnancy and Your Career

Your pregnancy and postdelivery period will affect your career, even if you decide to return to work soon after delivery. The Pregnancy Act of 1979 has helped women during pregnancy, and the Family Leave Act of 1993 has helped both mom and dad spend time with their child after delivery. However, every employer has individual policies regarding pregnancy and maternity leave. The following is a suggested list of questions to ask your employer/company regarding pregnancy and maternity leave:

1. How long may I continue to work while pregnant? If prolonged standing is required on the job, can another position be found for me after I can no longer stand for long periods? When I can no longer travel, can alternative work be found for me? Can alternative work be found if my doctor wishes me to cut back on my duties? Can I put in fewer hours if my doctor suggests it? Do you require the doctor to verify the safety of working during pregnancy?
2. Can I take leave before the baby is born? How soon? Do I get paid?

3. What is the company policy on maternity leave? Is this separate from vacation/sick leave?
4. Do I maintain my seniority while on maternity leave? Do I get paid while on maternity leave? Does the company consider maternity leave a disability?
5. Can I return to the same position? Is my job protected while I am on leave? For how long?
6. Is the maternity leave policy in writing? (If so, get a copy. If not, request it.)
7. How long do I have after birth before I must return to work? If a c-section is done, is that time extended? Can I take vacation/sick leave to stay home longer?

These questions need to be answered before you become pregnant. If you are having difficulty getting information or determining your maternity leave rights, consult the maternity leave resource guide in the appendices.

The Cost of Baby

Babies cost money, usually for the next twenty years or so. We will concentrate here on the initial costs and the impact on your finances. By using the following calculation sheets, you will find the approximate actual cost of having a baby, as well as the cost after the baby is born. As you will see, there are a lot of things to consider.

TABLE 1–1   *The Cost of the Baby*

COST OF LAYETTE*

	ONE TIME	MONTHLY
Bathing		
Clothing		
General needs		

TABLE 1–1   *The Cost of the Baby (continued)*

Safety needs   _____   _____

Linens   _____   _____

Total   _____   _____

BABY'S INITIAL TOTAL COST

Layette (total from above)   _____

Moving expenses (if applicable)   _____

Paint/wallpaper/nursery   _____

Childproofing   _____

Exercise classes   _____

Infant CPR classes   _____

Maternity clothes   _____

Prepared childbirth classes   _____

Maternal vitamins   _____

Obstetrician/caregiver fees**   _____

Special tests (e.g., sonogram, amniocentesis)**   _____

Genetic counseling (if applicable)**   _____

Hospital expenses**   _____

Anesthesia fees**   _____

Pediatrician fees (Newborn)**   _____

Circumcision (if applicable)**   _____

Total initial cost of baby   _____

*This is the initial cost. Some items, such as furniture, are more permanent. Other items, such as diapers and clothing are ongoing. Use the layette list in the appendices.

**Use the formula Initial Cost – Insurance Reimbursement = Actual Cost. Use the actual cost in your calculations.

TABLE 1–1   *The Cost of the Baby (continued)*

MONTHLY COST OF BABY

Monthly cost from
layette list above   _____

Well-baby care   _____

Nanny/day care   _____

Formula   _____

Total   _____ × 12 = _____ **Yearly**

CURRENT EXPENSES

	MONTHLY	× 12 =	YEARLY
Rent/mortgage	_____		_____
Telephone	_____		_____
Gas/electric/water	_____		_____
Transportation/car	_____		_____
Food	_____		_____
Entertainment	_____		_____
Clothing	_____		_____
Loans/credit cards	_____		_____
Investments/savings	_____		_____
Other	_____		_____
Total	_____		_____ **Yearly**

YEARLY EXPENSES WITH BABY

Current expenses   _____

Baby expenses (yearly)   _____

TABLE 1–1   *The Cost of the Baby (continued)*

Insurance	_____
Disability	_____
Life	_____
Medical	_____
Taxes	_____
Income	_____
Property	_____
Total Yearly Expenses	_____

TOTAL YEARLY INCOME

Self	_____
Partner	_____
Interest	_____
Dividends	_____
Total Yearly Income	_____

To determine your available yearly funds, subtract total yearly expenses from total yearly income. Enter here _____.

These calculation sheets will help you examine the cost of having a baby and its impact on your finances.

Now that the finances have been discussed and you have decided it is the right time to be pregnant, you need to be healthy and decide who will deliver your baby, and where and how you will deliver.

CHOOSING A PRACTITIONER

Family practitioners, certified nurse-midwives, lay midwives and obstetricians all deliver babies. One type of practitioner is not right for everyone; you need to make the choice on who is right for you. You can get ideas about who to use from friends, hospital referral services, birthing centers, telephone books, insurance carriers and advertisements.

Family practitioners are doctors whose practices encompass the whole family. They are primary care physicians who treat individuals as part of a family. Family practice is a relatively new medical specialty, yet it is a return to the way medicine was practiced for centuries before modern technology became available. Family practitioners have a three-year residency after medical or osteopathic school. At least three months of this time is spent in obstetrics and gynecology. The American Academy of Family Practice (or the American Osteopathic Board of General Practice) board certifies family practitioners and can verify this certification. (Addresses for these organizations are given in the appendices.) Not all family practitioners do obstetrics or are qualified in this area. Those that do, handle routine, uncomplicated obstetrics. If complications arise, they refer to obstetricians. Some hospitals require an obstetrician backup for privileges to be granted family practitioners for deliveries. Family practitioners also do not do operative deliveries.

Because they take care of the baby after birth, most family practitioners view childbirth as a normal part of family life. Like all practitioners, each is an individual in views and experience. It is your responsibility to find out about both.

Nurse-midwives are registered nurses who have had additional training in obstetrics for one to two years and have passed a certification examination given by the American College of Nurse-Midwives (see appendices for ACNM listing). They are then licensed by the individual states as to the scope of their practice. Nurse-midwives can be found in solo practice, in midwifery groups and in clinics and private OB practices. Nurse-midwives handle uncomplicated pregnancies and normal deliveries. Most of their deliveries are in hospital settings, with only about 10 to 15 percent at birthing centers. A very small number do home births. Nurse-midwives are not allowed to do operative obstetrics, although some are permitted to do episiotomies (the cut that can be made in the vaginal area to enlarge the opening), circumcisions and labor inductions. This varies from state to state. The majority of states require a written contract with a doctor for backup. The resurgence of nurse-midwives began in the 1950s and became prevalent in the seventies. It is your responsibility to discover the scope of midwifery allowed in your state. Your state department of health can direct you to the agency that will give you the information you seek.

Lay midwives practice in a home setting. They are not nurses and have no formal training. They apprentice by attending home births with an experienced midwife and help with the births. Some states do license lay midwives, but the laws vary so widely that you must check these for your state. If this is the practitioner you choose, you must check credentials, training and experience on your own since most are not regulated or licensed. Some lay midwives have delivered thousands of babies. The lay midwife may have a physician backup; you need to know this. You may have to arrange for backup medical care if it is needed.

Obstetricians are doctors who specialize in delivering babies. They have four years of college, four years of medical or osteopathic school and four years of internship/residency that is concentrated in obstetrics and gynecology. A relatively new subspecialty of obstetrics/gynecology is maternal-fetal medicine, which deals with high-risk pregnancies and requires an additional two years of concentrated training in obstetrics. Obstetricians are licensed to practice medicine by the state in which they practice. Most obstetricians are board certified by the American Board of Obstetrics and Gynecology. This board certification is considered to be the minimum standard of excellence and knowledge that an obstetrician should have. To verify whether your obstetrician is board certified, contact the American Board of Obstetrics and

Gynecology (listed in the appendices). A physician can be eligible to take the specialty boards for up to five years after completion of residency. This is called board eligible. His or her state license can be verified by calling your state department of health, which will direct you to the right agency for the information you seek.

The overwhelming majority of women choose an obstetrician to deliver their baby. At one time, obstetricians totally controlled the birth experience for mom, dad and baby. Times have changed, however. Now, families are able to choose how they want their birth experience to be. You have the right to choose a doctor who will listen to what you want. The first step is to interview him or her. The interview will answer the questions that are important to you and enable you to find a practitioner who is most appropriate. Do not expect doctors to know what you want. You must tell them what you want and ask if your wishes are feasible and in keeping with their philosophies. If you want the latest in technology and knowledge available, should it be needed, then an obstetrician may be the right choice for you. Obstetricians can handle any complicated pregnancy or any complication that may arise during delivery. There are many obstetricians who believe that childbirth is a normal, natural experience and do not treat pregnancy as a disease. They are not as rare as you might think.

Doctors perform an overwhelming majority of deliveries in hospitals; however, more and more are using birthing centers. Some still do home deliveries. If this is an option for you, you should be aware that not all malpractice insurance covers home deliveries. You must question the doctor as to which option is available to you.

Obstetricians may be in solo or group practices. Solo practices are becoming less common because of the demands of obstetrics. With a solo doctor, you will know, for the most part, who will deliver your baby. A group practice can have two or more obstetricians. In this type of setting, you may not be able to choose who will handle your prenatal care or who will deliver your baby; in-

TABLE 1–2   Pregnancy Caregivers—An at-a-glance look at each type of caregiver.

Caregiver	Education	Licensed	Training	Hospital Deliveries	Birthing Center Deliveries	Home Deliveries
FAMILY PRACTITIONER	Medical degree Osteopathic degree	In all states	3 years 3–6 months in OB	Yes	Yes	Yes* limited
LAY MIDWIFE	No formal training	In some states	Apprenticeship varies widely	No	No	Yes
NURSE–MIDWIFE	Associate in nursing Possible B.S.N., M.N.	In all states	1–2 years	Yes	Yes	Yes* limited
OBSTETRICIAN	Medical degree Osteopathic degree	In all states	4–6 years in OB	Yes	Yes	Yes* limited

*Malpractice insurance may not cover this. Please consult your caregiver.

stead, you will be seen by whoever is available. You need to question how each group handles a call schedule.

The Interview

To make a decision that will be the right one for you will take work on your part. You must interview the health care practitioners you are considering for your pregnancy needs. To determine philosophical agreement, you will also want to interview any backup doctors, nurse-midwives and lay midwives. The following list of questions will aid you in the search for the right practitioner.

PHYSICIANS
1. What undergraduate school did you attend?
2. What medical school did you attend?
3. Where did you do your residency?
4. Why did you choose obstetrics (family practice) as your specialty?
5. In what states are you licensed to practice?
6. Are you board eligible or certified?
7. Are you a member of the American College of Obstetrics and Gynecology (American Academy of Family Physicians)?
8. With what hospitals are you affiliated?
9. Do you deliver at birthing centers? Why or why not?
10. Would you consider home delivery? Why or why not?
11. What are your standard office hours?
12. Do you make house calls?
13. What is your protocol for taking phone calls?
14. Who covers your practice when you are unavailable?
15. What constitutes an emergency?
16. How are emergencies handled?
17. What are your views on prenatal testing, including chorionic villus sampling, amniocentesis and sonography?
18. What do you consider standard prenatal tests?
19. What do you consider a high-risk pregnancy?

20. Do you handle high-risk pregnancies? If not, do you have someone to refer to should a pregnancy become complicated?
21. What are your views on preconception counseling?
22. What are your views on fetal conditioning?
23. What is your stand on prepared childbirth classes?
24. What childbirth methods do you practice? Why?
25. In the event of a cesarean, are support people permitted in the operating room? Who does your cesarean sections?
26. Do you prefer labor, delivery and recovery in one room, or a labor room, delivery room and a recovery room?
27. When would you use forceps or suction in a delivery?
28. Do you allow the mother to breastfeed immediately?
29. Do you allow parent bonding immediately?
30. What percentage of your deliveries are cesarean?
31. What percentage of your deliveries involve episiotomies?
32. What is your view on circumcision?
33. Do you recommend prenatal vitamins?
34. When is labor induction a consideration?
35. Do you encourage birth plans?
36. How are financial matters handled? What is your standard range of fees? What insurance do you accept? Do you file insurance claims on patients' behalf?
37. Do you carry malpractice insurance?

CERTIFIED NURSE-MIDWIVES, LAY MIDWIVES

1. What nursing school did you attend?
2. What midwifery program did you attend (lay midwives: Where did you do your apprenticeship)?
3. Why did you choose to be a midwife?
4. How many deliveries have you done?
5. In what states are you certified (licensed) to practice?
6. When were you certified (licensed)?
7. Are you a member of the American College of Nurse-Midwives (lay midwives: Midwifery Alliance of North America)?

8. Do you deliver at hospitals? Why or why not?
9. Do you deliver at birthing centers? Why or why not?
10. Would you consider a home delivery? Why or why not?
11. What are your standard office hours?
12. Do you make house calls?
13. What is your protocol for taking telephone calls?
14. Who covers your practice when you are unavailable?
15. Who is your backup physician? Do I have to see him or her during my pregnancy?
16. Are you insured?
17. What constitutes an emergency?
18. How are emergencies handled?
19. What are your views on prenatal testing, including chorionic villus sampling, amniocentesis and sonography? Who does these procedures for you?
20. What do you consider standard prenatal tests?
21. Do you handle high-risk pregnancies? If not, to whom do you refer?
22. What do you consider a high-risk pregnancy?
23. What are your views on preconception counseling?
24. What are your views on fetal conditioning?
25. What is your stand on prepared childbirth classes?
26. What childbirth methods do you practice? Why?
27. In the event of a cesarean, do you attend the birth along with the physician backup?
28. Do you prefer labor, delivery and recovery in one room or separate rooms for each?
29. Would you use forceps or suction in a delivery? Are you certified for this?
30. What is your view on episiotomy? Are you certified to make and repair one?
31. What is your view on circumcision? Are you certified to perform one? If not, who would do it?
32. Do you recommend prenatal vitamins?
33. When is labor induction a consideration? Are you certified to induce labor? If not, who would do it?

34. How are financial matters handled? What is your range of fees? What insurance do you accept? Do you file insurance claims on patients' behalf?

After the interviews are completed, you should evaluate all the practitioners you have seen. Your choice is an obvious one. You want someone with whom you feel comfortable and who will allow your active participation in the pregnancy and birthing process.

WHERE TO GIVE BIRTH

Ninety percent of babies are born in hospitals, 8 percent in birthing centers and less than 1 percent at home. The remainder are born elsewhere and are attended by emergency medical workers, police officers, even cab drivers. Where you choose to have your baby (unless the baby has other ideas) is a decision you must make. Just as choosing a practitioner takes time and work, so does choosing the place you want to have your baby.

Hospitals

In a nationwide survey, we found hospital maternity care varies widely. Today, many hospitals are aware of what the public wants and try to comply. We found hospitals that still do deliveries only in delivery rooms. The majority of hospitals, however, have some form of birthing rooms available. We found hospitals that have some labor-delivery-recovery (LDR or birthing) rooms, along with traditional delivery rooms; some with LDR rooms with all operative deliveries (forceps, suction and C-section) being done in delivery rooms; some with LDR rooms that use delivery rooms for C-sections only. Hospitals often have combination rooms—labor-delivery-recovery (LDR, or birthing) rooms—along with traditional delivery rooms. Each hospital varies as to what is in the LDR room. You will find birthing rooms that are living room–

bedroom-type settings with all fetal monitors, IV apparatus, and so on, in the open or hidden and ready to be used on a moment's notice. You must visit the hospital yourself to see the type of facility available. This choice may be limited by the health care professional you choose to deliver your baby.

On your hospital visit, you must decide if it is in keeping with the philosophy you received from your doctor or midwife. Ask if rooming-in is allowed; how nurseries are used; if prepared childbirth classes are offered and what methods are taught; if breast-feeding specialists (sometimes called lactation consultants) are available to assist you; if the baby is taken from you at any time; if family-centered childbirth is a reality or an advertising phrase. You must also find out if you can leave in 24 hours if that is your choice.

Some hospital maternity areas are housed in separate but attached birthing centers located on the grounds of the hospital.

Birthing Centers

Freestanding birthing centers, physically separate from hospitals, are gaining wider acceptance. They are certified by the National Association of Childbearing Centers (see listing in appendices). Licensing is required in most states, but not in all. Birthing centers usually do no surgical deliveries, regional anesthesia or labor induction or augmentation. Freestanding birthing centers are usually backed by a hospital, where patients can be transferred if complications arise. Both doctors and midwives can deliver at birthing centers, but the majority of deliveries are done by midwives. Recent studies have shown that for selective patients (low-risk, normal pregnancies, especially in those women who have successfully had an uncomplicated vaginal delivery), a birthing center is an acceptable alternative. Birthing centers have fetal monitors and emergency equipment available. The safety of birthing centers is similar to hospitals, with about 15 percent of patients transferred to hospitals. The primary reason for such transfer is slow or stopped labor. Most of those transfers are first-time mothers. You must investigate the safety of the center you choose. Find out to which hospital transfers are made, how emergencies are handled and which doctors back up the midwives.

Home Birth

Home birth and home-style birthing centers and hospitals are not the same thing. Home births are not for everyone. For anyone with medical complications or a complicated pregnancy, this is not an option (see Table 1–3). Only those with the greatest possibility of success should choose home birth. Home birth requires planning and preparation, an experienced and qualified health care practitioner and an emergency transfer system in place should complications arise.

TABLE 1–3   *Contraindications for Home Birth as a Choice*

PREPREGNANCY PROBLEMS

Complications in a previous pregnancy
Age thirty-five or older having first baby
Delivery of six or more babies
Medical history of diabetes mellitus
Medical history of hypertension

PRENATAL PROBLEMS

Multiple babies
Hypertension that develops during pregnancy
Diabetes that develops during pregnancy
Rh incompatibility
Polyhydramnios
Placenta previa
Postdates baby

PROBLEMS DURING LABOR

Breech, transverse or other abnormal presentation
Pre-eclampsia, eclampsia

TABLE 1–3   *Contraindications for Home Birth as a Choice*
             (continued)

Cephalopelvic disproportion
Active Herpes infection
Premature delivery

The vast majority of home births are attended by lay midwives. Some nurse-midwives do attend home births, but this may be prohibited in your state. Doctors also may be restricted due to lack of malpractice coverage.

Again, the best way to decide if this is the birthing experience for you is to research and ask questions.

METHODS OF CHILDBIRTH

YESTERDAY AND TODAY

Jimmy dropped Betty off at the emergency entrance to the hospital and parked the car. When he finally found the maternity floor, he was told to wait in the fathers' room at the end of the hall. He would not see his wife again until the next day. Betty was admitted to an eight-bed labor room. An IV was started and she was given medication. When she was ready to deliver, the doctor was called. She was taken to a delivery room and strapped into stirrups. Forceps were used to pull out the baby. Betty was so drugged, that she did not realize until the next day that the baby was a girl. Dad, of course, knew; he had seen the baby behind the glass windows of the nursery. Jimmy took his wife and daughter home two weeks later, after an "uncomplicated" labor, delivery and recovery. That baby girl was ME.

Mary Jane went into the hospital for induction of labor after complications began in her pregnancy. She was placed in a private, single-bed labor room, where her support person stayed with her. After a long labor, she was taken into the delivery room and put in stirrups. She delivered a baby girl under bright lights and surrounded by people scream-

ing at her to push. Five days later, dad took his wife and tiny baby home. That beautiful baby girl was my DAUGHTER.

Christine was so excited—her pregnancy test was positive. The first thing she did was to call the physician she had previously chosen to deliver the baby. She and her husband made their first prenatal appointment and also registered for early pregnancy and nutrition classes. After these classes, they had to wait a month before they began Lamaze childbirth classes. These classes would train them to act as a team during the delivery. They also went to C-section classes on the chance that a surgical delivery would be necessary. They were glad they had. When the time came to have their baby, it was much too large to deliver vaginally. With dad at the head of the table beside her, Christine, awake with an epidural, was delivered via C-section of a beautiful baby boy. That little boy was MY GRANDSON.

Three generations and three very different childbirth experiences.

History of Prepared Childbirth

Before the 1920s, birth took place, for the most part, at home and was attended by doctors or midwives. In the twenties, women flocked to hospitals for the "new" modern methods of "painless" childbirth. This consisted of separating mom from the rest of the family, using drugs to make her oblivious to what was happening and creating a sterile environment for the newborn by separating mom, dad and baby. Breastfeeding was discouraged and was replaced with "modern" infant formulas and baby bottles. Soon, parents had absolutely no control over their childbirth experience; everything was orchestrated by the doctor. The natural, normal aspect of pregnancy no longer existed.

Not all doctors saw comatose childbirth as a positive step for mom and baby. Dr. Grantly Dick-Read in England saw the beauty in participatory childbirth. He noticed that women who had someone with them during labor to explain events had significantly less pain. In the 1930s he wrote *Birth without Fear*. Dr. Dick-Read was ridiculed by his American colleagues.

In the late forties, the Maternity Center of New York sponsored a grant to study the effect of Dr. Dick-Read's methods and to allow babies to "room-in." Fernande Lamaze, a French obstetrician, studied Russian techniques of conditioned response to reduce childbirth pain. His techniques were readily embraced by French women, who felt the American drugs were dangerous and expensive. Again, American doctors rejected his theories. However, two American women, Marjorie Karmel, who had her first child in Paris, and Elizabeth Bing, began a nationwide movement to promote the Lamaze method. The organization of the LaLeche League promoted a return to breastfeeding. In the sixties, Dr. Robert Bradley introduced the radical concept of fathers in the delivery room.

As women became more and more of a force in the marketplace and the workplace, their voices were heard. They began to demand participation in the childbirth experience.

Thus, today we have prepared, or "natural," childbirth. Prepared childbirth involves teaching methods to cope with normal childbirth and the natural sequence of events in labor and delivery. This gives mothers choices on how to have their babies and, along with their partners, allows them to make these choices based on information, not fear or ignorance. Even if they decide they want regional anesthesia, they will understand the effects on their bodies, as well as on their babies.

Prepared childbirth classes can encompass different aspects of the methods available today. My own practice uses this eclectic approach as well as incorporating many of my own ideas.

WHATEVER WORKS

Kathy was progressing nicely during the first stage of her labor. She and her husband, Ted, had prepared well. They remained calm and were using good breathing techniques. Kathy walked, rocked, showered and stayed mobile until she was about seven centimeters dilated. Since she had progressed so rapidly, she lost her focus and even with all our help was unable to regain it. She requested and was given an epidural.

Upon reaching complete dilation, she began pushing in a semi-sitting position. Ted coached her as she effectively pushed when her body told her. The epidural slowly wore off, and Kathy began to use the visualization-meditation techniques I had taught her to remain focused. After two hours of pushing, the baby seemed to want to stay where he was. Because Kathy was now in complete control, using breathing and meditation techniques, we decided to let gravity help deliver this stubborn child. With Ted sitting behind her and supporting her, Kathy held onto a bar over her head and squatted down. With me on the floor to guide the child into the world, Kathy delivered a beautiful baby boy. Ted reached over to cut the clamped cord. He helped Kathy to sit back on the bed and came to help me give the baby its first bath. As young Michael opened his eyes to the sound of his father's voice, he was wrapped in a towel. Michael met his mother when Ted placed him gently on her stomach. As mom, dad and baby got acquainted, the nurse was recording the birth events. After asking, the nurse was allowed to footprint the baby, give him vitamin K and place ointment in his eyes. All of this took place while Michael was on his mother's stomach. The new family was allowed to continue getting acquainted as my nurse and I left the dimly lit birthing room. As we were leaving, we heard the tinkle of the music box Michael had listened to while in his mother's womb.

A brief discussion of each method will give you an overview of each so that you can explore the method that appeals to you.

Lamaze

Lamaze is focused on control. By controlling breathing, you can control pain. By focusing on something other than the pain, you can control the pain or your perception of it. Exercises, as well as breathing techniques, are taught. Multiple types of breathing for various progressive steps of labor are covered so that attention is on breathing and muscle relaxation. All breathing starts with deep cleansing breaths. As contractions become more difficult, breathing may change. The coach's job is to monitor and help adjust the breathing pattern of mom. Pushing is accomplished by a deep, cleansing breath, followed by slow exhalation while pushing or holding the breath while pushing.

Bradley

Although challenged on being the only entirely natural childbirth method, proponents of the Bradley Method feel that there is danger in current obstetrical procedures. They disavow the safety of sonograms, episiotomy, and regional anesthesia. It is stressed that women are capable, and entitled, to give birth without drugs or medical intervention. They encourage the use of midwives rather than "technical-oriented" doctors. They further maintain that parents should take responsibility for the birth place, procedures and emergency backup.

Bradley teaches conditioning exercises and muscle relaxation. A slow, deep-breathing, take-your-time approach is advocated in a quiet, unlit, pillow-laden environment. Baby is immediately breastfed.

Kitzinger

Based on Dick-Read and Lamaze, the Kitzinger method employs mental imagery to enhance relaxation. The use of touch, massage and visualization helps the woman flow with the contraction rather than ignore or breathe it away. This method uses "puppet-strings relaxation," in which the partner tells the woman which limbs the strings are pulling, the others remaining relaxed. Long, slow, deep breathing is encouraged to achieve complete relaxation. Mom is encouraged to labor in any position that is comfortable for her; pushing is done when the body tells her it is time. Between pushes, short breaths are taken. The Kitzinger method emphasizes the empowerment of childbirth for women.

Gamper

The key to the Gamper method is the self-determination and confidence instilled by instructors in the ability of women to work and cooperate with the natural forces of childbirth. The emphasis is ON the contraction rather then AWAY from the contraction. A normal, natural rate of deep abdominal breathing is taught to help the woman work with the contraction. Classes begin early in pregnancy so that the fear-tension-pain cycle can be broken and new self-confidence instilled early on.

Simkins

The Simkins approach to childbirth works with the strengths of the couple giving birth. They are encouraged to use whatever means of breathing and style helps them as individuals. An eclectic mix of techniques is taught.

Noble

Elizabeth Noble's technique involves relaxation of the pelvic floor muscles. Her "gentle pushing," or "breathing the baby out" technique, is now incorporated in many classes. This approach encourages women to listen to their bodies.

LeBoyer

The LeBoyer method, introduced by French obstetrician Frederick LeBoyer in the 1970s, allows the baby to be born in a quiet environment amid dim lights and soft voices. It is given a warm water bath, then placed on the mother's abdomen for bonding. The newborn is handled gently and without sudden movement that may jar or startle it. LeBoyer babies open their eyes and breathe without being slapped on their bottoms. They smile, "talk" to mom and dad and move in a relaxed manner.

Because of this method's effects on newborns, hospitals no

longer allow loud, harsh noises in the delivery area. Babies are massaged at birth to begin breathing and not struck to begin startled, anguished cries.

Odent

Michael Odent, another French physician, went a step further than LeBoyer. He put mother and baby both in the water. Odent allowed laboring mothers to submerse in a pool of water. This appeared to help some women ease labor pain. When some of the women were reluctant to leave at the time of delivery, they were delivered in the water; the babies were unharmed since they had lived in fluid for nine months. The subsequent safety of this procedure has allowed the movement to be embraced in this country, and many centers and hospitals now have this option available.

Now that you've made your choices, it's time to start on a twelve-month journey that will change your lives.

✖ CHAPTER TWO

THE IDEAL TIMETABLE

Three Months before
Pregnancy

PREGNANCY AFFECTS EVERYONE

Now that you've decided to become parents, found your practitioner and chosen your birthing place, it's time to really begin.

Before you can become physically healthy to have a baby, you need to look at the emotions involved. Emotions influence your general health, body weight, relationships with others and other facets of your life. Pregnancy is a time of intense emotions for a woman, probably more so than at any other time in her life. Dad will also be feeling more emotional. You will both be bombarded by questions involving feelings. How will it feel to be parents, perhaps again? What will being pregnant be like? You will receive more advice than you have ever received in your life. Even strangers will come up to you and tell you how to feel. How will your parents, friends, coworkers and children feel about this pregnancy? What you need to understand is that *your* feelings are most important now.

Mom's body will change and become different. How this is perceived and reacted to by you and your partner will affect your interest in the pregnancy and each other. You need to know, before beginning, that pregnancy adds stress to any relationship. You need to trust each other, communicate your feelings, including your fears, and learn to compromise. No one ever said a pregnant woman was not emotional. Hormones have something to do with it, but even more important is the inner feelings you have about yourself and your partner. Body image can change sexuality, and your partner needs to be supportive of these changes.

25

Interest in sex can also be altered during pregnancy. Elizabeth Bing and Libby Coleman in *Making Love during Pregnancy* found four patterns: interest (1) increased throughout pregnancy, (2) increased in the middle trimester but decreased during the last trimester, (3) stayed the same, or (4) decreased throughout pregnancy. In other words, anything is possible. But with understanding and support, both mom and dad will be able to communicate their feelings.

As we progress through the weeks of pregnancy, we will address emotions that may be present during these specific times. Now it's time to get physically ready to have a baby.

PRECONCEPTION EVALUATION

Timing Your Visit

Both mom and dad should take part in the preconception evaluation. This should occur about three months before you plan to become pregnant. The length of the visit should allow enough time for mom to be examined, to have blood drawn for laboratory studies, to have both mom and dad's medical and family histories evaluated, and to have questions answered. A follow-up visit should be scheduled approximately one week later to go over the results. Let's review a basic evaluation.

Age

Age is important. Younger women have specific nutritional needs that must be addressed. Moms over the age of thirty-five can have an increased risk of genetic abnormalities and may be more at risk to develop complications in later pregnancy. Complications may be offset by proper nutritional preparation and more frequent visits throughout the pregnancy.

The age of dad also is important. There is now evidence that men over the age of fifty may have an increased risk of genetic ab-

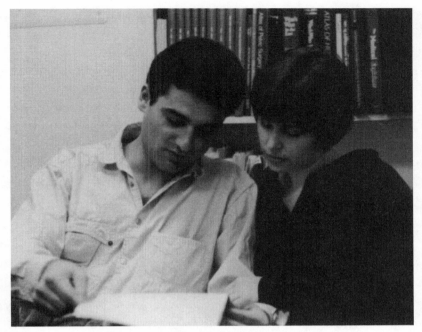

Having a baby is a couple decision.

normalities. Because the age of mom and dad is important, you need to be advised of the risks that may be encountered.

Marital Status

Having a significant other, whether a husband, lover or live-in friend, makes the pregnancy easier to cope with emotionally. Remember, this is a time of intense feelings. Your doctor needs to know the emotional support structure you have so that he or she can give your needs extra attention if the situation warrants.

Race

Certain diseases are more prevalent in some races than in others. Examples of this are Tay-Sachs disease in those of Eastern European Jewish heritage and sickle cell anemia in those of African descent. We will discuss this in more detail when we talk about family history.

Education

You should have on-going teaching throughout your pregnancy. Your doctor needs to be aware of your level of understanding so that he or she can communicate with you in language you understand. Whatever your educational background, however, your doctor should explain everything clearly and to your satisfaction.

Occupation: Past and Present

IT'S ONLY A COLD

Karen hadn't come in for preconception evaluation. During her visit at approximately four months into the pregnancy, she told me about a recent "cold." She hadn't bothered me because it didn't seem important at the time. What was important, though, was that she worked as a therapist with AIDS patients, many of whom had the virus CMV. This can give healthy patients a coldlike syndrome. I immediately ordered CMV titers. Of course, they came back extremely high. Some decisions now had to be made, because CMV infection during pregnancy can cause serious birth defects, including mental retardation. A follow-up titer had to be done in six weeks to see if this was a new infection; at that point, Karen would be past the fetal age for termination if she desired that. Karen and Joel, her husband, talked this over and decided to continue the pregnancy. However, they spent many a sleepless night over the next several months, until their beautiful, normal baby girl was born. All the anxiety had been for nothing and could have been prevented if they had come in for a preconception evaluation.

Occupational and environmental hazards need to be identified in both mom and dad. Exposure to lead, cadmium, PCPs and other metallurgic agents can affect sperm production and cause an increased rate of miscarriage. Exposure to solvents, lead, mercury and biologic and pharmaceutical agents can also affect the growing baby. You may need to monitor your exposure to such agents. For example, if you are a photographer and develop your own work, you may want to avoid color separations since agents in the developing solutions can affect the baby. If you are exposed to these agents, you may want to avoid them before trying to get pregnant.

The amount of physical exertion on the job is also a factor. If you are planning to get pregnant, you may want to modify your duties, such as lifting heavy objects.

A word about video display terminals: To date, studies have revealed no evidence that exposure to VDTs causes miscarriages or birth defects.

Your doctor should discuss these risks in detail with you.

Travel

If your job involves frequent traveling, you may have to limit it at the end of your pregnancy. Besides tiring you, travel can expose you to such diseases as malaria.

Pets

Animals carry diseases that can be harmful to the developing human baby. For example, cats carry a disease called toxoplasmosis that can affect the central nervous system of the developing fetus but not the adult who's infected. If you have a cat, your partner should change the litter box before the pregnancy, and you should be tested to see if you have ever had toxoplasmosis.

Habits

ALCOHOL

The effects of mom's alcohol use during pregnancy have long been recognized. Alcohol consumption by a pregnant woman can cause decreased growth before and after birth, specific facial abnormalities (such as low-set ears) and mental retardation (including learning disabilities and hyperactivity). These problems are all part of fetal alcohol syndrome (FAS).

More recent studies have shown that dad's alcohol use can also cause problems, including decreased growth before birth, learning disabilities, behavior problems and changes in the baby's immune system. These problems are called fetal alcohol effects (FAE).

There is no question that the mother's alcohol intake can cause the more severe problems. But in light of the recent findings about the father's consumption, refraining from alcohol should be done by both parents-to-be.

CIGARETTES

If mom smokes during pregnancy, she may have twice the risk of miscarrying. Decreased growth of the baby before birth has also been seen. Abruptio placentae (premature separation of the placenta from the uterus), placenta previa (the placenta covers the opening of the birth canal), premature rupture of the membranes (early breaking of the bag of fluid around the baby) and premature delivery have all been linked to smoking.

There may be an association between dad's smoking before pregnancy and an increased risk of brain cancer in the baby in later life, especially if the child is a boy. In addition, secondary smoke in the household or the workplace can increase the risk of minor learning disabilities. A recent study by the American Medical Association has shown that secondhand smoke gets to your baby. If you are around someone who smokes, your baby is "smoking."

Cigarette smoking should definitely be discontinued during

the preconception period. Consult your doctor about steps to take to stop smoking.

CAFFEINE

The use of caffeine has not been associated with birth defects of any kind. What may pose a problem, however, is substituting caffeinated drinks for proper food. Because caffeine is a stimulant that can affect the baby, mom may want to limit intake of caffeine to three or four servings a day, otherwise the baby may be break-dancing all night when you are trying to sleep. If you're a heavy caffeine user, you'll need to decrease your use gradually. The best time to begin is before pregnancy.

ILLEGAL DRUGS

The use of illegal drugs on either a recreational or an addictive level can be a big problem for your child.

Marijuana. Although the evidence is still not conclusive, enough questions exist that it is best to avoid using marijuana both before and during a pregnancy.

Cocaine. Cocaine and crack use by mom during pregnancy has been associated with heart and brain defects, learning disabilities, stillbirth, prematurity and decreased fetal growth. Crack use has been shown to cause abruptio placentae and an increase in the number of miscarriages.

The effects of cocaine use by dad is now being studied. There has been an association with learning disabilities in children born to fathers who used cocaine. Evidence exists that cocaine may attach itself to sperm and be carried to the egg during fertilization.

Because the effects can be devastating for your baby, illegal substance use should be stopped before you attempt to get pregnant.

Nutrition

The old adage "You are what you eat" can also be applied when preparing for your pregnancy. If you're not already practicing good nutrition, this is the best time to start. Moms who are more than 10 percent underweight can have babies who are smaller than they should be at birth. Moms who are more than 30 percent overweight have slightly larger than normal babies and are at an increased risk for complications in pregnancy, such as diabetes and high blood pressure.

Many women are deficient in iron, calcium, zinc and folic acid. Iron deficiency can cause mom to be anemic during pregnancy and put the baby at risk of anemia after birth. (Anemia is a condition that decreases hemoglobin, which is the blood component that carries oxygen throughout the body.) Zinc and calcium affect fetal growth, and folic acid is extremely important in the development of a healthy spinal cord. We now know that by giving women prenatal vitamins beginning three months before pregnancy, we can decrease the number of birth defects by 50 percent.

TABLE 2–1   *Weight Table for Women**

Height	Small Frame	Medium Frame	Large Frame
4'10"	92–111	96–121	104–131
4'11"	94–113	98–123	106–134
5'0"	96–115	101–126	109–137
5'1"	98–118	104–129	112–140
5'2"	102–121	107–132	115–143
5'3"	105–124	110–135	118–147
5'4"	108–127	113–138	121–151
5'5"	111–130	116–141	125–155
5'6"	114–133	120–144	129–159

*Adapted from the height and weight charts issued by the Metropolitan Life Insurance Company.

TABLE 2–1	*Weight Table for Women*		*(continued)*
5'7"	118–136	124–147	133–163
5'8"	122–139	128–150	137–167
5'9"	126–142	132–153	141–170
5'10"	130–145	136–156	145–173
5'11"	134–148	140–159	149–176
6'0"	138–151	144–162	153–179
6'1"	141–155	148–165	157–182

Your doctor should assess your nutritional status as part of your evaluation and begin prenatal vitamins. He or she should also make sure you are not taking megadoses of vitamins that could be harmful. These include vitamins A, C and D, which can all cause problems for your baby. If you are underweight, now is the time to gain; if you are overweight, now is the time to lose. Pregnancy is not the time to gain excess weight or to be on a weight reduction program. If you have specific dietary practices, such as vegetarianism or fasting, have food allergies or follow specific dietary laws, you need to discuss these with your doctor. You can use the prenatal evaluation form at the end of this chapter to begin.

Dad's nutrition is also important because he will want to eat a healthy diet in support of mom and for his own good health.

Tables 2–2 and 2–3 show the recommended daily requirements and various choices for a healthy diet.

TABLE 2–2	*Healthy Diet Choices**
Food Group	*Examples*
Protein foods	Fish, chicken, turkey, lean beef, eggs (whites), beans, peas, nuts
Leafy, green and yellow vegetables	Lettuce green peas, pumpkins, squash, yams, sweet potatoes, green and yellow beans, broccoli

Fruits	Oranges, tangerines, grapefruit, lemons, bananas, pears, apples, peaches, tomatoes
Other vegetables	Potatoes, brussels sprouts
Breads, cereals and flour	Cereal and breads, whole-grain crackers, pasta
Milk products	Low-fat milk, cheese, yogurt, ice cream

Current recommended daily servings for a healthy diet.

*Adapted from the Food and Drug Association's recent recommendations.

Avoiding empty calories now not only will help your baby when you become pregnant, but will help you get back to your prepregnancy weight faster. Avoid foods that are high in sugar and fat content. The better choices are high-fiber, low-fat, low-sugar foods. Use added fats, such as butter and salad dressings, in moderation. Begin eating healthy now so that your body can meet the demands of pregnancy.

TABLE 2–3   *Recommended Daily Servings*

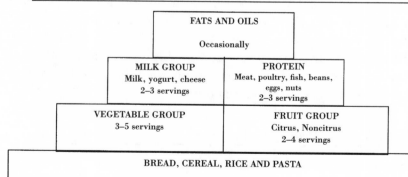

The new Food and Drug Administration daily recommendations for a healthy diet.

Exercise

Exercise is important for a healthy life. You should exercise a minimum of thirty minutes, three times a week. The exercise should be aerobic (raising your heart rate), such as brisk walking, running, low-impact aerobics, biking or swimming. Of course, other exercise may be done. As you near the time you are trying to get pregnant, you should practice keeping your heart rate under 140 beats per minute. You can take your pulse by placing your fingers on the side of your neck and counting the number of pulses for fifteen seconds, then multiply by 4. This gives your pulse rate per minute. If you do not exercise now, check with your doctor about the best way to begin. If you do exercise, great. Exercise during pregnancy is important and now is the time to start.

Stress

Continuous high-stress situations affect you and can affect your growing baby. If mom is under continual stress during pregnancy, the baby can stop growing or decide to make an early appearance. This doesn't mean that daily ups and downs will bother you or your baby; that's part of life. I'm talking about ongoing situations, such as deadlines, that cause stress for weeks or months at a time. You will want to assess your situation now so that problems do not occur later. You should also learn to relax now by practicing meditation, yoga, biofeedback or anything else that can help.

Sleep

Proper rest is important for your overall health. Humans need six to eight hours of sleep a day to function fully. If you have problems sleeping, talk to your doctor.

Family History

Because each of you contribute half of your baby's chromosomes (genetic material that determines specific features, such as eye color), your families histories are important. Hemophilia, Down's syndrome, mental retardation, sickle cell disease, muscular dystrophy and cystic fibrosis are all inherited. It is important that your doctor know if there is anyone in the family who has these or other hereditary problems. It is also important to know if there is a history of diabetes or high blood pressure in mom's family, since these can put her at an increased risk to develop these during pregnancy. Consult the form at the end of this chapter to evaluate your family history.

Medical History

Your past and current medical history is also very important. A record of childhood illnesses and immunizations for both mom and dad is essential. Contagious diseases such as rubella can be devastating during pregnancy. If you need immunizations, now is the time to get them. Some immunizations are safe during pregnancy (see Table 2-4). Dad can bring home measles and other diseases, so his immunization history is also important.

TABLE 2–4   *Immunizations During Pregnancy*

ALWAYS CONTRA-INDICATED

Smallpox
Rubella
Mumps & Measles
Hepatitis B

POSSIBLE CONTRA-INDICATIONS

Polio (Sabin-Oral)
Influenza

TABLE 2–4   *Immunizations During Pregnancy (continued)*

NEVER CONTRA-INDICATED

Yellow Fever
Plague
Tuberculosis (BCG)
Pneumovax
Rabies
Tetanus
Polio (Salk)

Any medications you are currently taking may need to be changed before pregnancy so that they do not affect your baby. An example is Coumadin, a blood thinner, which can cause birth defects. Heparin can be substituted. See Table 2–5 for other drugs that can cause birth defects.

Mom's current medical history is vitally important. Diabetes, high blood pressure, thyroid disorders, hepatitis and heart disease are examples of conditions that need to be handled with special attention in pregnancy both for mom's well-being and the baby's. Again, use the form at the end of this chapter to evaluate your medical history.

TABLE 2–5   *Drugs that Can Cause Birth Defects*

Androgenic steroids (Danocrine)

Anticoagulants (Coumadin)

Antithyroid drugs (PTU)

Anticonvulsants (Dilantin, Triidione, Depakene)

Lithium

DES

Chemotherapy drugs (Adriamycin)

Vitamin A isomer (Retin A)

Drug categories that can cause birth defects, with examples in parentheses.

Reproductive History

Both mom's and dad's reproductive history play a major part in determining a successful pregnancy. A history of miscarriages, pelvic infections or premature labor can affect the outcome, yet these are only some of the problems that can cause complications in the pregnancy you are now planning. Your past pregnancy histories and current and past forms of birth control are also important. If you are on the pill, now is the time to stop it. You need to have two normal periods before attempting to get pregnant. Use the evaluation form at the end of this chapter to do a detailed history. Be sure to ask questions specific to your health care.

Physical Examination and Laboratory Studies

Mom's physical assessment should include weight and nutritional status, blood pressure, heart rate and performance, thyroid evaluation (as part of hormonal health), lung capacity (asthma status), and abdominal (any abnormal growths), leg (varicose veins), breast (lumps or discharge) and pelvic (any fibroids, ovarian cysts, etc.) exams. Laboratory studies should include a test for anemia, kidney disease and cholesterol, as well as a Pap smear. Rubella immunity and any other diseases to which you may be vulnerable should also be ascertained. If you are at high risk (multiple sex partners, IV drug use), you should ask your doctor to do an HIV test. As many as half of all babies born to mothers with HIV are positive for the virus. TORCH titers may be drawn, to determine exposure to other diseases (T = toxoplasmosis, O = other, R = rubella, C = CMV, H = herpes and hepatitis).

After your examination and evaluation, your doctor will need to review the results and have you come back for recommendations.

LIFESTYLE CHANGES

Your doctor may make certain recommendations about your diet, exercise regimen, habits, vitamin use, medication changes and stress and exposure dangers. You will also start on prenatal vitamins.

In addition, your doctor may discuss specific tests that you will need during pregnancy, such as amniocentesis (a test that draws fluid from around the fetus to determine specific diseases and genetic problems).

Now may be the time to take a last fling or vacation as a couple. Remember, when the baby comes, you may find it a little more difficult to do mountain climbing for a while.

PREPARING THE WORLD

Now that you're preparing yourselves for the changes in your lives, you also need to prepare the people in your world. If you have children, you may want to begin talking about a new brother or sister. If changes have to be made in your job, now is the time to discuss this, as well as maternity/paternity leave, with your employer. You also need to know your rights as a pregnant worker. The time to find out is before you're pregnant.

Mom and dad are now healthy and prepared, but when is the best time of the month to get pregnant?

Preconception Evaluation

You and your partner should fill out the same forms, with the exception of the reproductive history.

Date: _____

Name: _____

Date of birth: _____ Age: _____ Race: _____ Sex: _____

Preconception Evaluation (continued)

SOCIAL HISTORY

MARITAL STATUS

Single _____ Married _____ Divorced _____ Widowed _____

EDUCATION   Last grade completed: _____

OCCUPATION

		POSITION HELD	NATURE OF WORK	# OF YEARS
Previous	1.	_____	_____	_____
	2.	_____	_____	_____
	3.	_____	_____	_____
Present	4.	_____	_____	_____

ANY EXPOSURE TO TOXIC/DANGEROUS MATERIAL?

	NO	YES	WHEN	NAME/TYPE	SYMPTOMS
Insulation	____	____	_____	_____	_____
Fumes	____	____	_____	_____	_____
Metal	____	____	_____	_____	_____
Chemical	____	____	_____	_____	_____
Plastics	____	____	_____	_____	_____
Solvents	____	____	_____	_____	_____
Dyes	____	____	_____	_____	_____
Animals	____	____	_____	_____	_____
Lead	____	____	_____	_____	_____
Radiation/ X-ray	____	____	_____	_____	_____

Preconception Evaluation (continued)

TRAVEL (LAST THREE YEARS)

		WHERE	WHEN
U.S.	1.	_____	_____
	2.	_____	_____
	3.	_____	_____
Foreign	1.	_____	_____
	2.	_____	_____
	3.	_____	_____

PETS   Cats _____ Dogs _____ Other _____

Do animals go outside? _____

Are animals immunized? _____

HABITS

	NO	YES	STARTED	STOPPED	AMOUNT	
Cigarettes	____	____	_____	_____	_____	pk/day
Coffee	____	____	_____	_____	_____	cup/day
Alcohol	____	____	_____	_____	_____	dk/day
Drugs	____	____	_____	_____	_____	

NUTRITION

MEALS   Regular   YES _____ NO _____ # Meals/day _____

#Snacks/day _____

Answer Yes or No to the following Questions:

YES   NO

____ ____   Always eat three meals a day

____ ____   Eat fewer than three meals a day

Preconception Evaluation (continued)

___ ___ Practice vegetarianism

___ ___ Eat dairy products and eggs

___ ___ Have fasted for longer than twenty-four hours

___ ___ Follow special dietary habits/laws

___ ___ Binge on any foods

___ ___ Vomit more than once a week

___ ___ Have eaten laundry starch, dirt or clay

Any food allergies? _____

What reaction? _____

Source of water supply? _____

EMOTIONAL STRESS

At Work: _____

Family: _____

Other: _____

EXERCISE

None _____ Irregular _____ Regular _____

Type: _____

_____

Sports Activities engaged in regularly: _____

SLEEP HABITS

Number of hours per night: _____

Time you go to sleep: _____

Time you awaken: _____

Do you use medications to fall asleep? _____

What do you use? _____

Preconception Evaluation (continued)

DRUG HISTORY

(List all drugs, including over-the-counter and illegal substances)

NAME	YEAR BEGUN	YEAR ENDED	REASON FOR TAKING	SIDE EFFECTS
1. _____	_____	_____	_____	_____
2. _____	_____	_____	_____	_____
3. _____	_____	_____	_____	_____
4. _____	_____	_____	_____	_____
5. _____	_____	_____	_____	_____
6. _____	_____	_____	_____	_____
7. _____	_____	_____	_____	_____

Have you ever taken illegal drugs? _____ Is yes, what? _____

When? _____ Last used? _____

ARE YOU ALLERGIC TO ANY MEDICATIONS?

NAME	YOUR REACTION
1. _____	_____
2. _____	_____
3. _____	_____
4. _____	_____

FAMILY HISTORY

Answer yes or no to the following questions:

YES	NO	
___	___	Twins
___	___	Italian, Greek, Mediterranean or Oriental background

Preconception Evaluation (continued)

___ ___ Hemophilia

___ ___ Jewish (Tay-Sachs Disease)

___ ___ Down's syndrome

___ ___ Mental retardation

___ ___ Sickle cell disease

___ ___ Muscular Dystrophy

___ ___ Cystic fibrosis

___ ___ Huntington chorea

___ ___ Three or more miscarriages

___ ___ Diabetes

___ ___ High blood pressure

___ ___ Tuberculosis

___ ___ Short stature

___ ___ Large babies (over ten pounds)

___ ___ Birth defects (heart, spine, etc.)

If yes, what kind? _____

MEDICAL HISTORY

CHILDHOOD

(Check if you have had any of the following)

___ Mumps	___ Whooping Cough	___ Kidney Disease
___ Measles	___ Scarlet Fever	___ Pneumonia
___ Rubella	___ Rheumatic Fever	___ Heart Murmur
___ Chicken Pox	___ Nephritis	___ Mononucleosis

Preconception Evaluation (continued)

IMMUNIZATIONS

(Enter the date)

____ DPT (Tetanus)   ____ Polio   ____ Measles

____ Mumps   ____ Rubella   ____ Flu

____ Pneumococcal   ____ Hepatitis

Check if you have or have ever had any of the following:

____ High blood pressure   ____ Diabetes

____ Kidney disease   ____ Heart disease, including
                                 MVP

____ Thyroid disorders   ____ PKU

____ Hepatitis   ____ GI disorders

____ Neurologic disorders   ____ Tuberculosis

____ Urinary tract disease ____ Mental illness

____ Multiple Sclerosis   ____ Epilepsy

____ Collagen vascular disease, including lupus, rheumatoid
     arthritis, scleroderma

____ Blood transfusion

     If so, when? _____

____ Cancer, other than breast or genital tract

____ Asthma

ANY SURGERY?

	DATE	WHERE	WHAT
1.	_____	_____	_____
2.	_____	_____	_____
3.	_____	_____	_____

Preconception Evaluation (continued)

ANY HOSPITALIZATIONS?

	DATE	WHERE	REASON
1.	_____	_____	_____
2.	_____	_____	_____
3.	_____	_____	_____

ANY SERIOUS ACCIDENTS?

	DATE	ACCIDENT
1.	_____	_____
2.	_____	_____

REPRODUCTIVE HISTORY (MOTHER-TO-BE)

Check if you have or have ever had any of the following:

_____ HPV (Condyloma)   _____ Gonorrhea

_____ Genital herpes   _____ Syphilis

_____ Abnormal Pap   _____ Ovarian cancer

_____ Breast cancer

_____ Pelvic infections

If so, when? _____

Check if the answer is yes to any of the following questions:

_____ Have you had Rh sensitization in a pregnancy?

_____ Have you had a tubal pregnancy?

_____ Have you had any pelvic surgery? If so, what?

_____ Have you had any genital tract surgery?

_____ Did your mother take DES when she was pregnant with you?

_____ Is there a family history of breast cancer?

_____ Is there a family history of ovarian cancer?

Preconception Evaluation (continued)

Have you ever had any of the following:

____ Two or more abortions over fourteen weeks

____ A miscarriage over sixteen weeks

____ Three or more miscarriages

____ A c-section

____ An infant weighing more than nine lbs.

____ An infant weighing less than five lbs.

____ Any premature deliveries

____ Any fetal deaths

____ Any infants with birth defects

____ Any premature labor in previous pregnancies

Pregnancy History

Have you ever been pregnant? _____

How many times? _____

Have you ever had problems in a previous pregnancy? _____

Details _____

Have you ever had problems getting pregnant in the past? ___

Details _____

Menstrual History

Age at first menstruation _____ Regular _____ Irregular _____

Days between onset _____ Days duration _____

Number of pads per day _____ Last menstrual period _____

Birth Control History

Have you ever used an IUD? _____ When? _____

Why removed? _____

Preconception Evaluation (continued)

What type was it? _____

Have you ever used oral contraceptives? _____ When? _____

Name _____ Discontinued _____

What is your current method of birth control? _____

Date of Last Pelvic Exam: _____ *Last Pap:* _____ *Results:* _____

REPRODUCTIVE HISTORY (FATHER-TO-BE)

Check if the answer is yes to any of the following questions:

_____ Have you had any genital tract surgery?

_____ Did your mother take *DES* when she was pregnant with you?

_____ Have you ever fathered a child?

_____ Have you ever fathered a child with a birth defect?

_____ Do you wear bikini briefs?

_____ Do you wear tight jeans?

If so, how often? _____

_____ Do you regularly use a jacuzzi?

_____ Do you regularly use a sauna?

CHAPTER THREE

OPERATION: CONCEPTION

Two Months before
Pregnancy

THE RIGHT TIME

Georgina was a fashion designer for a new company, and Peter traveled a great deal in his position as a civil rights attorney. They had stopped using birth control about a year ago and were still not pregnant. They came to see me, sure that something was wrong. Their preconception evaluation revealed that Peter was away from home frequently, often three weeks at a time. When queried about the times of the month they made love, they revealed that it was whenever they were together. Sometimes, that togetherness was not at the right time of the month. I advised them to consider altering Peter's travel schedule, which didn't seem possible. I also suggested that Georgina accompany him on trips, which also wasn't always feasible. The last suggestion I made was that they take a well-timed vacation together. Two months later they came in for their first prenatal visit. They assured me it was the relaxation and timing of the vacation that did it.

EMOTIONAL TIMING

The pressure is on! That's the way many couples feel. You've made the decision to get pregnant, you're healthy and prepared. The performance stress you put on yourself can sometimes work against you. The best thing to do is relax and enjoy each other. Once you know the time of the month that you can get pregnant, make love at that time. Don't expect to get pregnant in any one month; give yourself six months. That will ease the pressure.

SEX   CHROMOSOMES

FEMALE   **MALE**

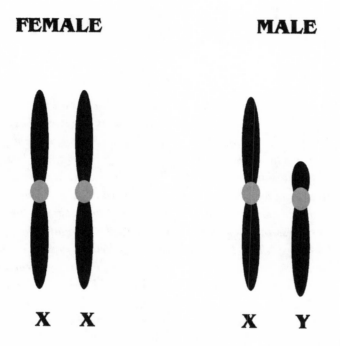

X   X   **X   Y**

From the instant of fertilization, the sex of the baby is determined.

PHYSICAL TIMING

Each human being's genetic structure is made up of forty-six chromosomes (twenty-three pairs). One half of these come from the mother and the other half from the father. Two of these chromosomes determine the sex of the baby. From the instant of fertilization (joining of the egg and sperm), the sex of the baby is determined. The egg always carries one X chromosome. The sperm carries either an X or Y chromosome (the father determines the sex of the baby). Two X chromosomes will result in a female; an XY combination will result in a male.

THE FEMALE ANATOMY AND HOW IT WORKS

FEMALE ANATOMY, FRONT VIEW

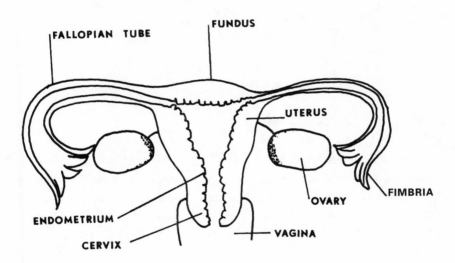

Ovum, or eggs, are stored in the ovaries. Two ovaries are located in the pelvis, one on each side of the uterus. The ends of the fallopian tubes have fingerlike projections called fimbria that grab an egg when it is released (ovulated). The fallopian tubes are connected to the uterus (the organ where the baby grows). The lower opening of the uterus, the cervix, is located at the top of the vagina.

All the eggs a woman will ever have are formed while she is still in her mother's uterus. These five million eggs have already formed by the time the mother is five months pregnant, and this

FEMALE ANATOMY, SIDE VIEW

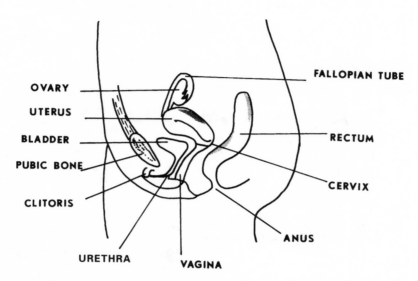

OVARY

UTERUS

BLADDER

PUBIC BONE

CLITORIS

FALLOPIAN TUBE

RECTUM

CERVIX

ANUS

URETHRA   VAGINA

number is reduced to half a million by birth. Any infections or toxic substances that can cross the placenta while the mother is pregnant can affect this baby's future childbearing. However, this will not be known until she is ready to have a child of her own. An example of this is DES exposure, which has affected a whole generation of women.

Girls are beginning menstruation at an earlier age than a century ago due to better nutrition. There is a set amount of body fat that is needed for menstruation to begin, and because girls generally weigh more today, they are menstruating earlier.

Every period starts a cycle that usually produces a single egg that can be fertilized. Cycle lengths vary from twenty-one to thirty-five days, but are usually twenty-eight days in length from the beginning of one period to the beginning of the next. An area of the brain signals the pituitary gland (a tiny gland located at the base of your brain and above the roof of your mouth) to produce the hormones FSH and LH. These hormones are then

MENSTRUAL CYCLE

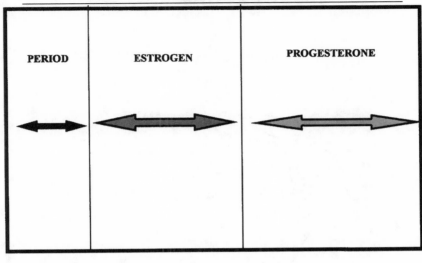

| PERIOD | ESTROGEN | PROGESTERONE |

DAY   5   14

The average menstrual cycle is twenty-eight days. Ovulation occurs fourteen days from the beginning of your next period. The first part of the menstrual cycle is when estrogen is produced. After ovulation, progesterone is produced.

released into the bloodstream, where they are conveyed to the ovaries. Stress, grief, trips or anything that disrupts a woman's life can keep FSH and LH from being released, thus causing lack of a period.

FSH and LH reach the ovaries and signal them to produce the female hormone estrogen. Estrogen signals an egg to begin to ripen. The egg is ripened in a sac called a follicle. When the egg has completely ripened, it is released from the follicle into the abdomen, where it is picked up by the fimbria of the fallopian tubes.

Ovulation, which takes only about two minutes to complete, usually occurs fourteen days after the onset of the period in a twenty-eight-day cycle. Ovulation always occurs fourteen days before the onset of your period. Thus, if you have a thirty-five-day cycle, you will ovulate on day 21 (see Table 3–1).

The egg is capable of being fertilized for twenty-four hours. If

OVULATION

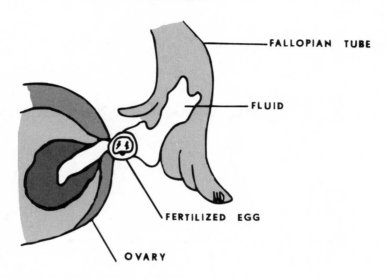

fertilization doesn't occur, the egg dies. A small amount of bleeding can occur with the rupture of the follicle. This can produce a discomfort called mittelschmerz.

A woman can detect the approach of ovulation by a change in her cervical mucus. It becomes more watery and is present in larger quantities. This helps the sperm move through the mucus on its journey to the egg awaiting in the fallopian tube.

The follicle, or sac that housed the egg before ovulation, now begins to produce a hormone called progesterone, which is sent into the blood. Progesterone causes changes to occur in the lining of the uterus, the endometrium, which will allow the fertilized egg to nest or implant. Progesterone also causes changes in cervical mucus, making it thicker and thus unable to be traversed by sperm or bacteria.

If fertilization does not occur, the lining of the uterus is shed, resulting in a period.

Women ovulate approximately 400 times from puberty to menopause. All the eggs not ovulated by menopause have died.

Ovaries also do not necessarily take turns in releasing eggs. If one ovary is surgically removed, the remaining ovary will produce an egg a month.

THE MALE ANATOMY AND HOW IT WORKS

MALE ANATOMY, SIDE VIEW

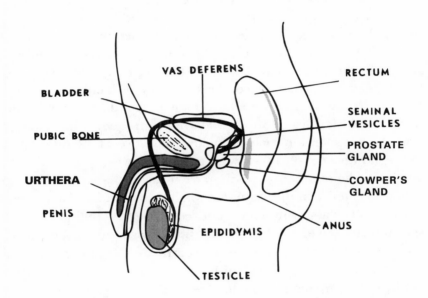

The testes (plural of *testis,* or *testicle)* are where sperm are formed. The new sperm travel through the epididymis, behind each testicle, where they mature. The mature sperm travel through a tube called the vas deferens through the seminal vesicle, a sac near the bladder. In the seminal vesicle, semen is added. The semen-sperm mixture (ejaculate) passes through the prostate and joins the urethra. The ejaculate travels through the urethra (the tube that carries urine from the bladder to the end of the penis) and is discharged.

Contrary to women, who produce an egg a month, men are capable of producing billions of sperm. Even though the numbers can decrease after the age of forty, men are capable of producing sperm from puberty well into later life. Men can be fathers in their eighties and nineties.

Men are born with immature sperm cells called spermatogonia. At puberty, the pituitary gland produces the exact same two hormones, FSH and LH, that it produces in women. However, the effect in men is very different. One causes the testes to produce the male hormone testosterone, which is required for sperm to mature and for the sex organs to become fully operational. A healthy young man can produce about 1,000 sperm per minute, and they are produced in the part of the testes called the seminiferous tubules. Each ejaculation contains roughly 500 million sperm. However, about half of these have some defect that render them incapable of fertilizing an egg. The more frequent the ejaculation, the less sperm in each ejaculate. Therefore, at the right time of the month a couple might want to make love every other day to maximize the number of sperm in each ejaculate.

Sperm can live in the vagina, cervix, uterus and fallopian tubes for up to five days. Only a few hundred of the 250 million healthy sperm reach the egg. It takes about two hours to make the entire journey to the egg; however, some sperm are Olympic swimmers and can reach the egg in a half hour.

The sperm are made capable of fertilizing an egg by substances found in the cervix, uterus and fallopian tubes. If no egg is available to fertilize, the sperm swim around patiently waiting for one. Because there is no chemical or physical attraction of the sperm for the egg, the sperm literally must bump into the egg.

WHEN CAN YOU BECOME PREGNANT?

An entire menstrual cycle is measured from the first day of your period to the first day of your next period. Ovulation occurs fourteen days *before* your next period. Table 3–1 gives the probable day you should ovulate, based on the length of your cycle. Because the egg lives for twenty-four hours, sperm need to either be there to meet it or arrive shortly after ovulation. By making love on alternate days, the production of sperm will be at peak levels each time.

For a twenty-eight-day cycle, you should make love on days 11, 13, 15 and 17. Remember, sperm can live up to five days. By following this schedule, sperm will always be present in the right place.

TABLE 3–1   *Probable Ovulation Day*

Length of Cycle	Day of Ovulation
21	7
22	8
23	9
24	10
25	11
26	12
27	13
28	14
29	15
30	16
31	17
32	18
33	19
34	20
35	21

Ovulation occurs fourteen days BEFORE your period starts. Your cycle is counted from the first day of your period to the first day of your NEXT period.

TABLE 3–2   *Basal Body Temperature Chart*

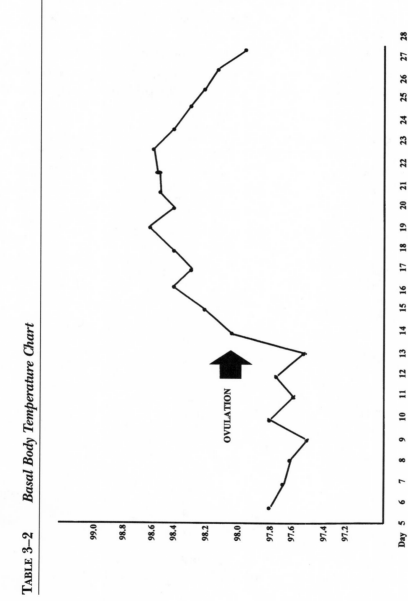

The basal body temperature chart can help you determine when you ovulate. Take your temperature each morning before getting out of bed and mark it on the corresponding day. When your temperature goes up several tenths of a degree, you are ovulating.

Basal Body Temperature

A woman's body temperature varies throughout her menstrual cycle. This temperature variation is mediated by the hormones progesterone and, to a minor extent, LH. You can use this information to predict ovulation. Using a special thermometer, called a basal body thermometer, you must take your temperature every morning *before* getting out of bed and record this in the chart that comes with the thermometer. Your temperature will begin to rise on day 13 of a twenty-eight-day cycle and continue to rise until approximately day 15. From day 15 until a few days before your period, it will remain elevated. If you're pregnant, it will remain elevated. If you're not pregnant, your temperature will begin to decline.

Ovulation Predictor Kits

Ovulation predictor kits work by detecting the small amounts of LH present in the urine before ovulation. There is a rise in the amount of LH in the body approximately twenty-four hours before ovulation. This increase is registered by a color change. You must follow manufacturer's directions precisely to get the best results.

Now that your ovulation day has been established, it's time for the sperm to meet the egg.

CHAPTER FOUR

THE SPERM MEETS THE EGG

Getting Pregnant

HOW CONCEPTION OCCURS

Before ovulation occurs, the fimbria (fingerlike ends) of the fallopian tube are positioned over the ovary (see illustration on page 52). These fimbria move along the ovary until a follicle containing the ripened egg is found. The lining of a fallopian tube contains millions of hairlike projections, called cilia, that move back and forth creating suction. When ovulation occurs, this suction sweeps up the egg, along with some of the fluid that has surrounded the egg in the follicle. The chemicals in the fluid signal the muscles of the fallopian tube to contract. These contractions propel the egg gently toward the uterus.

After the egg is in the fallopian tube, it continues to ripen and prepare itself for the sperm. The egg is surrounded by a nourishing shell that the sperm must penetrate. Each of the hundreds of sperm work hard to penetrate the shell, layer by layer. Suddenly, one sperm breaks through the shell and instantly a chemical reaction takes place, making it impossible for any other sperm to penetrate. The area of the egg containing the mother's genetic contribution (chromosomes) and the area of the sperm containing the father's combine to begin a brand-new, unique individual. About twenty-four hours after fertilization, the first division of the newly formed cell takes place. The dividing ball of cells continues to travel down the fallopian tube toward the uterus.

FERTILIZATION

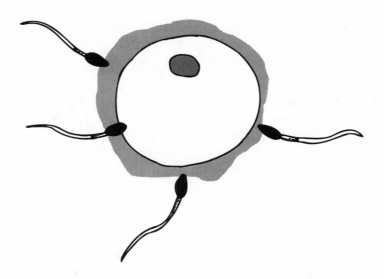

HOW LONG SHOULD YOU TRY TO GET PREGNANT?

About 85 to 90 percent of couples will get pregnant within one year. After the age of thirty-five, this rate declines for women. There is a further decrease for women after the age of forty. As mentioned earlier, sperm production for men decreases after the age of forty.

PROBLEMS ACHIEVING PREGNANCY

A couple may have a fertility problem if they do not achieve pregnancy after one year of unprotected intercourse. At one time, it was assumed that it was the woman's "fault" if she did not become pregnant. Now we know differently. The subject of infertility, the inability to get pregnant, would fill many books this size; here, we will discuss it briefly.

Whose "Fault" Is It, Anyway?

Male	40%
Female	40%
Both	5–10%
No Reason	10–15%

At one time women were believed to be at fault if conception did not occur. We now know that 40 percent of the time the male partner has a problem, 40 percent of the time the female partner has a problem, 5 to 10 percent of the time both partners have a problem and 10 to 15 percent of the time no reason can be found.

Male Problems

ABNORMAL SPERM

A decreased number of sperm can contribute to infertility. A count of 20 million sperm per milliliter is considered normal. When examined microscopically two hours after a sample is obtained, 50 percent of the sperm should be moving and 60 percent should be of normal shape.

ANATOMIC ABNORMALITIES

Developmental problems, such as failure of the testes to descend at the appropriate age and abnormal formation of the testes, epididymis, vas deferens or urethra, can all contribute to infertility.

TOXINS/DAMAGE/DISEASE

Infections such as tuberculosis, syphilis and gonorrhea can cause damage to structures that convey the sperm. Mumps, surgery and traumatic injuries can cause an inability to produce sperm. Radiation, chemicals and various drugs (both legal and illegal) could also contribute to infertility.

HEAT

Regular use of saunas, hot tubs and Jacuzzis can increase the temperature of the testes, thus not allowing an adequate number of sperm to be produced.

An abnormality in the size of veins in the scrotum, called a varicocele, can also cause an elevation in temperature. A varicocele is a weakening of the wall of the vein, much like varicose veins seen in the legs.

BIRTH DEFECTS

Defects in formation of any of the sex organs can cause infertility. There has been some evidence that DES sons can have structural defects.

ABNORMAL SEMEN

Semen, the seminal fluid that mixes with the sperm, may be too thick. The normal amount of semen in a single ejaculate is between three and five centimeters. Too little may not allow sperm to be separated enough to swim, and too much may dilute the concentration of sperm.

ANTIBODIES

Antibodies are formed to fight disease in the human body and work by sending messages to the white blood cells. The white blood cells then destroy the bacteria or other substances. Rarely, the body makes antibodies against sperm, and the sperm are then attacked by the white blood cells.

OTHER

Impotence, premature ejaculation (ejaculating before the penis enters the vagina) and retrograde ejaculation (backup of sperm into the bladder instead of through the urethra) can be factors preventing pregnancy.

Female Problems

NO OVULATION

Because signals from the brain to the hypothalamus to the pituitary must be perfect every month, the possibility exists that there may be an interruption of this process. Without these signals, nothing notifies the ovaries to make estrogen and progesterone, and ovulation does not occur. The interruption or error can happen one time or on a continuing basis.

An increased amount of estrogen can keep ovulation from occurring. Progesterone also has to be produced in the correct amount or the lining of the uterus will not be ready for the embryo (the fetus in the first eight weeks after conception) to implant.

TUBAL DYSFUNCTION

Sexually transmitted diseases, earlier IUD use and scar tissue from previous surgery can all cause tubal dysfunction. The tube must be open and able to pick up the egg at ovulation. Endometriosis is a problem for 10 to 15 percent of women. The question of how much endometriosis contributes to infertility is still unanswered. What is known is that the effects of endometriosis can cause infertility. These include tubal closure, pelvic scar tissue and inability to ovulate.

UTERINE ABNORMALITIES

An abnormal shape, previous surgery or scar tissue inside the uterus will not allow the fertilized egg to properly implant. DES daughters can have abnormally shaped uteri.

CERVICAL ABNORMALITIES

Cervicitis, an inflammation of the cervix, can interfere with sperm crossing the cervix on the way to the uterus. Previous cervical surgery, such as cautery, cone biopsies or cryosurgery, can cause abnormalities in cervical mucus. There is a condition called hostile cervical mucus in which white cells or antibodies in the mucus kill the sperm.

OTHER

Using lubricants to facilitate intercourse can create an unfavorable environment for sperm and they will die. Pain during lovemaking, which does not allow complete penetration, can interfere with fertility.

A last mention of timing is in order. In order to become pregnant, fertilization must occur during the appropriate period in your ovulation cycle.

No reason for infertility will be found in 10 to 15 percent of couples unable to conceive.

A BASIC INFERTILITY EVALUATION

A basic infertility work-up should include a semen analysis and a basal body temperature review. The semen analysis will assess the amount, shape and mobility of the sperm. If any abnormality is present, the man may be referred to a urologist for a complete evaluation. The basal body temperature review will establish if and when ovulation is occurring.

To see if the sperm and cervical mucus are compatible, a postcoital test can be conducted. The couple makes love at home, then the woman is examined in the doctor's office. The procedure involves a vaginal speculum examination and extract of some of the cervical mucus. The mucus is examined for estrogen content and sperm movement, shape and numbers.

The next step is to make sure that the amount of progesterone is correct. This is assessed by taking a small amount of the endometrium and examining it under a microscope. The day of ovulation can be predicted within twenty-four hours. If this is out of sync, an abnormal amount of progesterone is being produced. Your doctor can give you progesterone vaginal suppositories to correct this problem.

Laboratory studies can assess if you are making the right amount of hormones.

Tubal patency is assessed using an X-ray examination called a hysterosalpingogram. Radio-opaque dye is injected into the uterus through the cervix. This is conveyed through the fallopian tubes if they are unobstructed.

Even though the condition is rare, a test is done for antisperm antibodies.

If no other cause is found for the inability to conceive, the last step of the infertility evaluation may be a laparoscopy. This is a surgical procedure that involves maneuvering a small telescope-like device through the umbilicus (the navel or belly button) to examine the pelvic structures.

After your infertility evaluation is complete, your doctor will inform you of what steps can be taken to correct the individual problems.

ALTERNATIVE METHODS

Twenty years ago, if you could not get pregnant, your options to have a child were limited to adoption. That is not the case today. A brief description of alternative methods to achieve pregnancy follows.

Artificial insemination allows the couple with a sperm or cervical mucus incompatibility problem to conceive. Either the partner's sperm or donor sperm can be used.

In vitro fertilization (IVF) was developed in the 1970s. The first successful "test tube baby," Louise Brown, was born in 1978. Since that time technology has improved greatly. IVF involves removing an egg from the woman's ovary and fertilizing it in a special solution outside the body using a semen specimen. After the fertilized egg reaches a certain number of cell divisions, it is returned to the uterus. About 25 to 30 percent of couples can achieve pregnancy with IVF.

WE DID EVERYTHING

Carol and Doug had been trying to get pregnant for several years. They came to me for an infertility evaluation, but a work-up showed no indication of any problems. I referred them to a leading IVF center as candidates. They were aware that it could take up to six attempts before pregnancy was achieved. After completion of the first cycle of IVF, Carol came to see me because she had not had her period when it was due the week before. She was anxious to begin the second IVF cycle and wanted to be sure that nothing was wrong. After an examination and pregnancy test, I was happy to tell Carol that she did not have to return to the IVF center: She was pregnant. The thought had never entered their minds that they would be successful on the first attempt. Carol was so excited that she called Doug from my office. She was crying so hard that she couldn't talk. I had to tell Doug myself that he was going to finally be a father. It wasn't until I introduced them to their son, Frederic, eight months later, that they finally believed they were really going to be parents.

Gamete intrafallopian transfer (GIFT) involves removing an egg from the woman's ovary, mixing it with sperm and placing the mixture into the fallopian tube where fertilization will hopefully take place. Zygote intrafallopian transfer (ZIFT) is similar to IVF. The fertilized egg is placed at an earlier stage into the fallopian tube. Donor egg pregnancies use the IVF technique. The egg, however, is donated from a woman who will NOT carry the fetus. All of these techniques require a specialist in reproductive endocrinology/infertility.

Now that conception has occurred, let's discover that you're pregnant.

🌺 CHAPTER FIVE

YOU'RE PREGNANT? YOU'RE PREGNANT!

First Month of Pregnancy

🌺 HOW DO YOU KNOW WHEN YOU'RE PREGNANT?

Many times, mom will just *know*. It may be a feeling or sense that you get that a new life has begun. Sometimes mom has symptoms of pregnancy.

SYMPTOMS OF PREGNANCY

All the symptoms of pregnancy (see Table 5–1) are the result of the combination of two hormones, progesterone and human chorionic gonadotropin (HCG). HCG is excreted almost immediately after the tiny group of cells has implanted in the endometrium. This hormone tells the ovaries that pregnancy has occurred and no more ovulations are needed. The ovaries, in turn, now make more progesterone. Some women are extremely sensitive to hormone changes in their bodies and will have symptoms of pregnancy very early. However, most symptoms of pregnancy become evident between the fourth and eighth week of gestation.

TABLE 5–1   *Symptoms of Pregnancy*

Fatigue	Breast tenderness
Frequent urination	Breast enlargement
Heartburn	Mood swings

TABLE 5–1   *Symptoms of Pregnancy (continued)*

Nausea   Headaches
Vomiting

You may notice these symptoms even before you have missed your first period. Most of these symptoms, however, will not show up until after the fifth week.

I CAN HANDLE THIS; I'VE READ ALL THE BOOKS

A thirty-eight-year-old patient, who had been trying for two years to get pregnant, called on the Fourth of July because her period was a day late. She wanted a pregnancy test done immediately, and I arranged one for her. The test was positive and the patient came into the office the following week with her husband for her first prenatal visit. She was feeling absolutely wonderful. She had invented pregnancy and was ready to take on the world.

One week later, at six weeks, this dynamic woman called because she had spent the past three mornings hovering in the bathroom, afraid to move, due to waves of nausea. She asked how she could possibly continue to manage her company, of which she was CEO. All she was doing now was running out of meetings, nauseous from the smell of coffee and cigarettes.

She told me she was managing a billion dollar company and yet she had no control over her own body. The romance of the pregnancy had obviously worn off. She looked terrible, she stated; she couldn't even put on makeup. She slept almost twelve hours a day, yet she was still very tired. She said that she couldn't take this for another eight months and wanted to speed up the pregnancy, that it wasn't what the books had said. Her body felt invaded. Her husband was ready to kill her, because she had the most unreasonable mood swings. He wanted to send her to a spa until the baby was born.

About four weeks later, the symptoms had passed and again she felt elated. All was wonderful. In the end, she gave birth to a beautiful baby boy.

HOME PREGNANCY TESTS

Today's home tests are very sensitive and can detect a pregnancy as early as ten days after conception. A chemical in the test kit reacts with HCG to indicate the presence of the hormone. To get accurate results, be sure to follow product directions.

YOUR FIRST PRENATAL VISIT

You and your partner should schedule a prenatal visit as soon as you think you're pregnant.

The hospital or birthing center you have chosen will receive copies of the prenatal records you will complete on your first visit. These records will contain personal information about both of you, your medical and family histories and your physical examination. In addition, the birthing site will receive a copy of your complete prenatal care history.

Physical Examination

Your physical examination should include assessments of your heart, lungs, abdomen and pelvis. The pelvic examination may help to confirm your pregnancy (see Table 5–2). Your doctor should also evaluate your pelvis and do specific measurements to assess if it is adequate to deliver vaginally. Your weight and blood pressure should be recorded. Blood should be obtained for syphilis; blood type; Rh and blood antibodies; a complete blood count, including hemoglobin, hematocrit and white blood cell count; and glucose and hepatitis B. Some patients ask for an HIV test to be done. If you wish this done, you should ask your doctor now if you have not done so at your preconception examination. Urine should be checked for glucose and protein. A test for tuberculosis should be done.

TABLE 5–2   *Diagnosis of Pregnancy*

SIGNS OF PREGNANCY

Missed period   "Blueing" of vaginal mucosa
Skin changes   Skin discolorations
Breast changes

EVIDENCE OF PREGNANCY

Increased size of the uterus   Softening of the cervix
Softening of the uterus   Positive pregnancy test

ABSOLUTE PROOF OF PREGNANCY

Detection of fetal heartbeat   Ultrasound visualization of fetus
Fetal movement

Your health care practitioner makes the diagnosis of pregnancy
based on many factors.

Your doctor will set the length of times between visits. Usually,
you are seen every four weeks until the twenty-eighth week; then,
every two weeks until the thirty-sixth week. During the last weeks
of pregnancy you will be seen weekly.

Due Date

Your doctor will give you an expected due date based on the date
of your last menstrual period. To get a close calculation, subtract
three months from your last menstrual period and add seven
days. A normal pregnancy lasts 266 to 294 days. This equals forty
weeks, or ten lunar months.

Diet and Weight Gain

You should already be on a healthy diet, but now that you're pregnant, you'll need to increase your intake by 300 calories a day to gain the proper amount of weight. You should thus consume 2,100 to 2,400 calories a day. You also need to consume seventy-five to eighty grams of protein a day. Avoid liver, however, since reports have shown that liver contains levels of vitamin A that may be toxic to your baby. Fish is an excellent source of protein, but make sure that it is fresh and not high in iodine. Your calcium intake should be 1,200 milligrams a day. This can be obtained from dairy products. If you cannot tolerate dairy products, your doctor may recommend a calcium supplement. Divide your calories so that an evening snack becomes a regular part of your daily nutrition, and make sure you have two servings of food containing vitamin C.

You will consume enough natural fats if you follow the diet recommendations. Trim excess fat from foods. Use lean cuts and steam, bake or broil meats. Use olive oil rather than vegetable oils. Use low-fat dairy products, but avoid skimmed milk. The ma-

TABLE 5–3   *Recommended Daily Servings during Pregnancy*

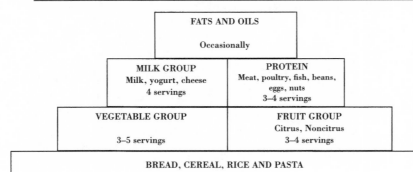

Recommended daily servings for a pregnant woman to maintain a 2,100- to 2,500-calorie diet.

jority of your calories should be carbohydrates. Avoid empty calories such as those in cakes, cookies, potato chips, soft drinks, sweetened juices and candy. (I recommend that my patients avoid artificial sweeteners, even though no harmful effects have been attributed to these additives.) It is also important to drink at least eight glasses of water a day.

One-Serving Equivalents

PROTEIN

3 ounces lean red meat, fish, chicken, poultry

3 eggs

4 ounces soft cheese

12 ounces yogurt

4 ounces shrimp

1/4 cup peanut butter

3 ounces hard cheese

1 cup dried beans

MILK GROUP

1 cup of milk

12 ounces yogurt

2 ounces hard cheese

3 ounces soft cheese

1 1/2 cups of ice cream

2 cups of cottage cheese

FRUIT GROUP

4 ounces citrus juice*

3 ounces strawberries*

1 large lemon or orange*

1/2 medium grapefruit*

9 ounces tomatoes*

1/2 cantaloupe, mango, papaya

1 medium apple

1 medium banana

VEGETABLE GROUP

1 ounce green, yellow pepper*	1 medium potato
1 cup broccoli, carrots, brussel sprouts, cauliflower, kale, sweet potatoes, spinach	1 cup asparagus

BREAD, CEREAL, RICE AND PASTA

1 slice whole grain bread	1 whole grain tortilla
3 ounces brown rice, bulgur, kidney beans, chickpeas	3/4 cup cooked cereal
	3/4 cup pasta
6 whole grain crackers, breadsticks	3/4 cup dry cereal

FATS AND OILS

Occasionally

*Vitamin C sources

A healthy pregnancy weight gain is twenty-five to thirty-five pounds. This is all accounted for by the pregnancy and the changes in mom as a result of the pregnancy. The usual weight gain distribution is five to seven pounds the first thirteen weeks, ten to fourteen pounds the second thirteen weeks, and ten to fourteen pounds the last thirteen to fourteen weeks.

If you're still not gaining enough weight, your doctor may add calories to your diet. I recommend the following:

Nutritious Milkshake Recipe

1 1/2 cups low-fat milk	1 small banana
1/2 cup cooked oat cereal	1/2 cup strawberries
1 tablespoon wheat germ	Honey to taste

Combine all ingredients and blend until desired thickness is obtained. This is good for a nighttime snack as well as for breakfast. You can keep cooked oats in the refrigerator for two days. I suggest patients add this milkshake to their daily diet if weight gain is not sufficient.

In addition, you should continue to take your prenatal vitamins.

Exercise

With some modification, your regular exercise program can be continued during pregnancy, although your heart rate should not exceed 140 beats a minute. Exercise for thirty minutes, three times a week. Because your oxygen consumption increases during pregnancy, the intensity of the exercise should be modified. You must make sure that you are adequately hydrated at all times. Stop exercising when you become tired. *Do not push yourself to your prepregnancy limits.* Always precede and end each workout with a warm-up and cool-down period of at least five minutes each.

Deep flexing and extension movements should be avoided. Because of hormone changes, joints become lax during pregnancy and you may hurt yourself. You may continue weight training; however, decrease amounts and limit the strain on your joints. Avoid exercises that involve deep knee bends and "bearing down." Jumping, jarring and bouncing movements should be avoided. Competitive sports, such as singles tennis, may need to be curtailed. Do not do exercises on your back after the fourth month. Full, strenuous activity should continue for no more than fifteen minutes at a time. As you progress through the months of pregnancy, your doctor should modify your exercise regimen.

Drugs During Pregnancy

Before taking any drugs during pregnancy, you should review them with your doctor. This includes over-the-counter medications. Any drug you take can affect your baby.

YOUR EMOTIONS

Mom

Even though you have planned for this pregnancy, the reality of it may be overwhelming to you. You have so many thoughts and they all seem scattered in different directions. You may worry about how you'll look as the pregnancy advances, what will happen if you have complications, how long you'll be able to work, how do you know you really want a baby, how this will really affect your personal relationships or how you'll handle labor. All of these thoughts may hit you at one time. Relax. It's normal to have conflicting emotions during pregnancy. A lot of this is hormone related. You will begin to think more and more of your baby as the pregnancy progresses.

We'll discuss the most common emotions for each stage as we progress through the pregnancy.

Dad

Right now, the pregnancy doesn't seem quite real to you. Your partner may have started to have mood swings and cry for no apparent reason. The thought of really being a father may be terrifying. You may not even believe it, even though you have planned for it. As irrational as the thought may be, you may even wonder how you could be the father. This is normal. You may be excited, fearful and anxious all at the same time. You may even wonder if you're being replaced by this unseen child. You could have fears that something could happen to your partner. These thoughts and feelings decrease as the pregnancy progresses and becomes more real. Women become more involved at the beginning of a pregnancy, but you can become involved by understanding your partner's mood swings and expecting them. You can become more nurturing by giving gentle massages and indulging her. This may make you feel more a part of things. Go with her to the prenatal visits. This is your baby, too.

Because your concerns can be different from your partner's, we'll talk about your emotions as we progress through the pregnancy.

WHAT YOUR BABY LOOKS LIKE

The First Few Weeks

The weeks of pregnancy are counted from the last menstrual period, even though we know that conception occurs approximately two weeks after the beginning of that period. Normally, a pregnancy lasts from 266 to 294 days.

Generally during weeks 1 to 4, the last two weeks are the weeks since conception. Because of the confusion, we will always refer to the age of the baby in number of weeks since your last period. To describe what is happening during the crucial first two weeks, we will talk about hours to days since fertilization. During this time, you may have an idea that you are pregnant, but most symptoms are yet to come. Your missed period may be the first real sign that a new life has begun. Many changes have occurred since that fused or joined egg and sperm divided to form two cells.

The fertilized egg remains in the fallopian tube approximately three days. It continues to divide as it makes its way into the uterus. If the fertilized egg does not make it to the uterus, the result will be a tubal pregnancy.

One crucial journey has ended and another is about to begin. The fertilized egg has become a hollow ball of cells called a blastocyst. The blastocyst must now find a place in the uterus to nest or implant.

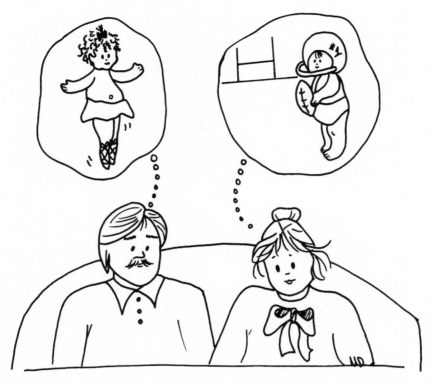

Mom and Dad each have their own ideas about the baby.

The blastocyst nestles in the endometrium approximately seven days after fertilization and begins to release the hormone HCG into the mother's blood. The endometrium, changed by the hormones HCG and progesterone, is ready to receive the blastocyst. The area where implantation occurs is changed the most. Blood vessels come to the surface of the endometrium. These will be used to exchange the nutrients and oxygen from the mother's blood to the growing fetus, through the placenta. Each cell of the blastocyst is now unlike any other. These differentiated cells will form all parts of the fetus and placenta.

Crucial developments have occurred during the first few weeks after conception: fertilization, the joining of the sperm and egg; travel down the fallopian tube to the uterus; nesting or implant-

THE FIRST WEEK

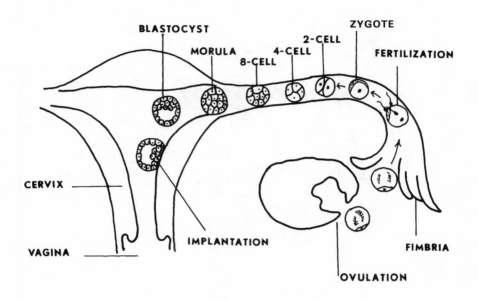

ing in the uterine lining; the beginning cell divisions; and formation of the placenta. This is an extremely crucial time for the embryo in which the slightest defect in the interplay of cells can lead to severe malformations. This interplay can be affected by the mom's daily life, habits and intake of drugs or medications that can interfere with the cells doing their proper jobs. Nature, in its infinite wisdom, has built-in safeguards. If the damage is severe enough, the pregnancy will end in miscarriage, sometimes before mom is even aware she is pregnant.

SOME OF THE THINGS YOU CAN EXPECT

"Morning sickness" can occur at any time of the day. It may occur by the fourth week and usually lasts until the twelfth or thirteenth

IMPLANTATION

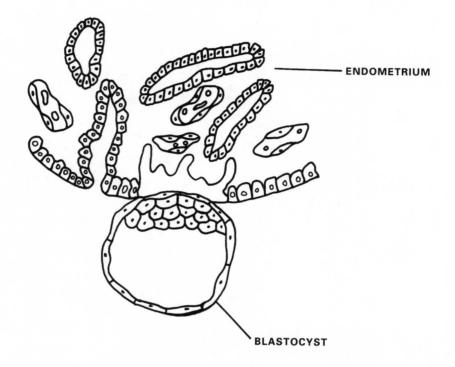

ENDOMETRIUM

BLASTOCYST

week. Occasionally, it extends beyond the thirteenth week. Because everything you eat is rapidly turned to glucose to feed the developing fetus, you can develop low blood sugar. Women who are more sensitive to low blood sugar may experience nausea. Sensitivity to pregnancy hormones also plays a role in morning sickness. Unlike the nausea associated with an illness, the nausea of pregnancy increases when the stomach is empty. To avoid this,

1. Eat frequent small meals.
2. Eat dry crackers or dry toast before getting out of bed in the morning.

3. Drink peppermint or rose hip tea during the day, between meals.
4. Avoid fatty, fried or spicy foods.
5. Keep areas well ventilated both at home and at work.
6. Get out of bed slowly in the morning.
7. Avoid long periods without food.
8. Chew on five or six anise seeds between meals.

Constipation occurs because food goes through the digestive system at a slower pace due to the effects of progesterone. Progesterone relaxes smooth muscle; therefore, food is propelled more slowly by the smooth muscle of the intestines. As food slows down, more water is absorbed from the contents of the colon, creating a harder stool. Iron, in your prenatal vitamins, can also contribute to constipation. Drinking more water and eating more fiber may help. You should *not* take laxatives. If constipation becomes a problem, ask your doctor to recommend a natural stool softener.

Fatigue is caused in part by the sedative effect of progesterone. Your body will tell you how much sleep you need. Learn to listen.

Frequent urination at this stage of pregnancy is the result of increased kidney function to rid the body of waste products and toxins. Your kidneys are now working for two—you and your baby. You may want to avoid regular hot and iced teas. Tea has a natural diuretic effect. A better choice would be herbal tea. Drink plenty of fluids, especially water, to replace what you lose.

Heartburn is caused by progesterone's relaxation of the smooth muscle at the entrance of the stomach. This allows a backflow of the contents of the stomach into the esophagus. The esophagus reacts to the stomach acid, producing a burning sensation. Antacids may relieve this, but get your doctor's advice on which one to use.

Breast changes in early pregnancy are the result of vessel engorgement. Vessels in the breasts become enlarged because of smooth muscle relaxation. The smooth muscles in the veins relax, which in turn causes the valves located in the veins to work less efficiently. This results in the vessels' becoming engorged with blood. Wearing a good support bra, properly fitted, will help. If your breasts are large, wearing a bra while sleeping may be beneficial. If you have breast implants, check with your doctor concerning the advisability of breastfeeding.

Faintness/dizziness is caused by a decrease in the flow of blood to the brain. This happens because more blood is going to the uterus and because the smooth muscles of the veins are relaxed, causing pooling of blood in the legs. Low blood sugar can also contribute to faintness/dizziness. You can avoid this by changing your body position slowly (lying to sitting, sitting to standing) and by not standing in one position for long periods. Eating frequent, small meals may also help. If you do feel faint, sit down immediately. If sitting does not help, lie down or put your head between your legs.

Mood swings and apprehension are the result of both pregnancy hormones and your own variable and changing feelings about being pregnant. Talking with your partner or a friend, a gentle massage, reassurance that this is normal and meditation may all help.

Meditation should calm and relax. To meditate, go to a quiet place, if possible. Close your eyes and relax all your muscles slowly, starting with your toes and working your way up your body. Take deep, slow breaths as you relax the muscles of your body. Imagine yourself floating on a white cloud. Slowly allow this cloud to envelop you, so that you are surrounded by calm, white light. As the white light surrounds you, visualize your baby growing within you, healthy and happy. In your thoughts, talk to your baby. Continue the slow, deep, calming breaths as you open your eyes, refreshed and relaxed.

Headaches can be common throughout pregnancy. They may be caused by tension, low blood sugar, mild dehydration or vascular effects of hormonal changes. Eating frequent small meals, drinking plenty of fluids, and employing meditation and relaxation techniques may help. You should *always* inform your doctor about headaches.

Cramps are not uncommon in early pregnancy. Mild, menstrual-like cramps happen to some women. If they become severe or persist for long periods of time, notify your doctor immediately.

Skin changes can occur during pregnancy. Although most changes occur later in pregnancy, some can be apparent very early. These include acne, dryness, pigmentation changes, spider veins, blotchy skin and increased sensitivity to cosmetics. Raised estrogen levels cause the spider veins and blotchiness. Along with estrogen, increased levels of progesterone and melanocyte-stimulating hormone (MSH), a hormone that is responsible for skin pigmentation, cause an increase in skin pigmentation. This is more pronounced in women with dark hair. The increased levels of hormones can also cause increased oiliness or dryness of the skin. Every woman is different, and there is no way to predict how the hormone changes will affect you. Using natural moisturizers, facial cleansers and cosmetics may help.

Hair becomes thicker and grows faster as a result of hormonal changes. Normally, you lose 15 to 20 percent of your hair at any one time. During pregnancy, this rate of hair loss decreases to 10 percent. You may also react to hair color or dyes. Avoid the fumes and unpredictability of metallic dyes and ask your hairdresser to use natural vegetable hair products. Permanents are unpredictable during pregnancy.

Nails also grow faster during pregnancy. Splitting and breaking can occur. Keep nails short and use hand creams liberally.

Your vision may be affected. During pregnancy the cornea of the eye thickens as a result of water retention. If you wear contact lenses, you may find yourself less able to tolerate them. Some women experience vision changes very early in their pregnancy.

Vaginal discharge increases normally in pregnancy due to the rapid turnover of cells. It should be white, odorless and nonirritating. You may be more comfortable wearing a panty liner if your discharge is copious. If the discharge becomes very thick, cottage cheese–like, odorous or itchy, call your doctor. Yeast infections are very common during pregnancy and should be treated by a doctor. Remember, even simple things should be handled differently during pregnancy.

Sleep disturbances can occur even in early pregnancy. The increased metabolism you are now having as well as the thermogenic effects of progesterone will cause an increase in body heat. Frequent urination may force you to get out of bed several times a night. Heartburn happens throughout pregnancy and can be more intense at night, when you are lying down. As the pregnancy progresses, the increase in abdominal pressure may exacerbate the general discomfort you feel. Disturbing dreams also can occur throughout pregnancy. These are common and normal. You may have dreams that you will miscarry, that something will be the matter with your baby or that you will have problems with labor and delivery. These dreams mean nothing and are not portents of things to come. Some of the things you can do to improve your sleep is meditate, have a gentle massage in the evening, drink camomile tea at bedtime and use an antacid one hour before going to bed. Experiment with "white" noise (sounds of oceans, winds, rain) in your bedroom and sleep with your head and shoulders elevated on extra pillows or a special pregnancy pillow. Also, be sure not to have any caffeinated drinks after 3:00 P.M.

COMPLICATIONS THAT CAN OCCUR

Ectopic Pregnancy

An ectopic pregnancy is a pregnancy in which the fertilized egg implants outside the uterus, usually in a fallopian tube. The number of tubal pregnancies has increased in recent years.

Call your doctor immediately if you experience severe lower abdominal pain with or without bleeding. This is a medical emergency and you need to be examined as soon as possible.

ECTOPIC PREGNANCY

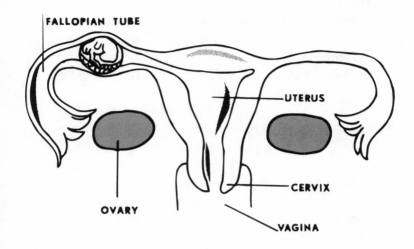

FALLOPIAN TUBE

UTERUS

OVARY

CERVIX

VAGINA

Hyperemesis Gravidarum

Some women experience severe nausea and vomiting during pregnancy. This is called hyperemesis gravidarum. Frequent vomiting episodes should be reported to your doctor. You can quickly become dehydrated and lose electrolytes, which are necessary to keep your body functioning properly. If you are unable to keep anything in your stomach for more than twenty-four hours, you should notify your doctor.

Miscarriage

A miscarriage is the loss of a pregnancy. About 25 to 35 percent of all pregnancies end in miscarriage, with 75 to 90 percent of all miscarriages occurring in early pregnancy, sometimes before the woman even realizes she is pregnant. The reasons can include genetic problems in the fetus, infection, hormonal imbalance and incompatibility between the mother's and father's blood types (an example of this is a mother who is Rh negative and has antibodies to Rh positive blood, which the father may have). The medical term for miscarriage is *spontaneous abortion*. A spontaneous abortion is preceded by bleeding about 95 percent of the time. Bleeding, however, does not necessarily indicate that a miscarriage will occur. The bleeding may or may not be accompanied by cramping.

A spontaneous abortion can be classified as one of the following:

1. A *complete abortion* involves expulsion of all products of conception, including the fetus and placenta.
2. A *habitual abortion,* which involves more than one pregnancy, has occurred at the same time in at least three pregnancies. An example of this is multiple miscarriages midpregnancy due to an incompetent cervix (the cervix opens prematurely).
3. An *incomplete abortion* is one in which only part of the products of conception are expelled.
4. An *inevitable abortion* is one in which the cervix has opened. This is usually accompanied by cramping.
5. A *missed abortion* occurs when the fetus and the placenta die but are not expelled. There may be no bleeding with a missed abortion.
6. A *recurrent abortion* is one that has occurred at least three times, at a different time in each pregnancy and for different reasons.
7. A *threatened abortion* is one in which bleeding occurs but does not progress to loss of products of conception.

QUESTIONS

1. Is sex safe?

Sex is safe during pregnancy as long as there is no bleeding, ruptured membranes or history of premature labor. You may have to adjust positions for comfort as your pregnancy advances.

2. Is oral sex safe?
Yes, as long as your partner does not blow into the vagina, since air could enter the bloodstream.

3. Can I use a microwave?
Yes, microwave ovens have safety shields built in. If the oven does happen to leak, you would have to stand directly in front of it for a long period of time for any harm to occur.

4. Can I go through airport detectors?
Airport metal detectors are not harmful to you or your baby.

5. Can I fly during early pregnancy?
You can fly during pregnancy with some precautions. You should get up and move around every hour, drink at least one liter of water for each two to two and a half hours in flight and try to keep your legs elevated as much as possible on very long flights. I ask patients not to fly domestically after thirty-four to thirty-six weeks, internationally after thirty-two weeks. If you must fly after thirty-two weeks, take copies of your medical records with you.

6. May I go to the dentist during pregnancy?
Good dental care should continue throughout pregnancy. Advise your dentist that you are pregnant and avoid any unnecessary X rays. You should have your dentist call your doctor before administering any anesthetics or medications.

❧ CHAPTER SIX

WHY DO I FEEL SO LOUSY IF I'M SO HAPPY?

Second Lunar Month of Pregnancy

PHYSICAL CHANGES

Your body is undergoing tremendous changes. Many are a continuation from the beginning of pregnancy, and others are occurring for the first time during this month. Morning sickness may worsen and nausea may happen at any time. You may develop an aversion to certain smells, such as brewing coffee, or certain foods and drinks that you loved before pregnancy, such as milk. You may become increasingly tired and may sleep twelve hours a day. Spider veins, thin veins at the surface of the skin, may begin to show on your thighs. If you have varicose veins, they may begin to bother you more. Your breasts will continue to increase in size, due to the expanding milk ducts, and be tender. Dark blue veins may begin to show through the skin on your breasts. The areola, or area around the nipple, begins to darken. Frequent urination is becoming normal.

EMOTIONAL CHANGES

Mom

You may notice a decreased interest in sex because of fatigue and nausea. Mood swings are becoming more prevalent, ranging from joy at being pregnant to depression at being pregnant, sick, tired and scared. You begin to think more and more about your baby and its well-being.

Dad

Dad deal with the symptoms of pregnancy in many ways. Some became frightened that their partners are "sick." Others become frustrated that the pregnancy lasts so long. Your own partner may fear losing you as you become preoccupied with the pregnancy, or may even become "pregnant" with you. Couvade syndrome is a phenomenon in which men show the symptoms of pregnancy, including morning sickness, weight gain, loss of appetite and fatigue.

WHAT CAN WE DO FOR MORNING SICKNESS

Sarah and Jason had planned for their baby and had come in for pre-conception counseling and evaluation. Jason was very excited about becoming a father and couldn't wait for them to be pregnant. They became pregnant four months after evaluation. At the first prenatal visit, Jason asked more questions than Sarah did.

About two weeks later, Sarah called the office in a panic. The vomiting had been unrelenting for two days. What could be done? My secretary immediately put her through to me, afraid that Sarah had developed hyperemesis gravidarum and needed to be hospitalized. Upon questioning Sarah, I learned that she was handling the nausea and had no vomiting. She had called about Jason, who had developed more pregnancy symptoms than she had. I prescribed a medication to help with the vomiting, and Jason was fine the next day. He did continue to be nauseous, but the vomiting ceased.

YOUR PRENATAL VISIT

You should see your doctor about four weeks after the initial visit.

What Should Be Done

Weight

Blood pressure

Urinalysis for protein and glucose

Discussion of any problems or questions you both may have (be sure to write down any questions when you think of them)

WHAT YOU SHOULD BE DOING

Even though you're tired most of the time, try to exercise. It'll make you feel better. Don't push yourself and don't feel guilty if you can't exercise as much. If you have varicose veins or a family history of varicose veins, you should start wearing support panty hose, avoid standing for prolonged periods and exercise.

Start thinking about your maternity wardrobe; you'll need it sooner than you think. You may notice that your clothes are already becoming snug and that you're more comfortable in loose clothing. Pay attention to your increasing breast size. It may change rapidly, and you need to wear well-fitted bras.

Travel may be difficult due to fatigue and nausea. Plan ahead and travel when you have the fewest symptoms. Motion sickness can be a problem now, even if you've never experienced it before.

Eat whatever foods you can. Frequent small meals are better than three large ones.

If you have children, you may want to tell them about the baby if you're experiencing a great deal of morning sickness. Children become frightened when they see that their mom is ill. Depending on the age of each child, you should explain that the symptoms you have are normal.

YOUR BABY

During the period between the fifth and eighth week, the embryo, what your baby is now called, grows from eight-hundredth of an inch to a half inch in length. It has changed from a hollowed ball of cells to what appears to be an almost humanlike being. All of the organ systems are formed by one of three cell layers, called germ cells. The outer germ cell layer forms the brain, nerves, spine, skin, hair and sweat glands. The middle layer forms the blood cells, blood vessels, heart, ovaries, testes and kidneys. The stomach, intestines, lungs and bladder are formed from the inner germ cell layer. The developing organ systems are coordinated with each other, but they are not fully functioning at this time.

The placenta is working to shunt blood, carrying oxygen and nutrients through the umbilical cord vein to the baby. Waste products from the baby are carried back to the placenta through two umbilical arteries. Any drugs taken by mom may now go directly to the developing baby through the placenta. The yolk sac, which forms the blood cells at this time, and the fetal side of the placenta are between the membranes surrounding the embryo. The outer membrane, the chorion, and the inner membrane, the amnion, will fuse later in the pregnancy. The yolk sac will disappear and the fetal liver, spleen and bones will take over its job.

At five weeks of pregnancy, the heart tube begins beating and pumping blood to the aorta and developing liver. At six weeks, the quarter-inch-long embryo has begun forming a brain and spine. The face, arms and legs start to grow in the sixth to seventh week. Fingers and toes are beginning to be seen. The tip of the nose is clearly distinct.

At eight weeks, the spinal cord is clearly visible through the transparent skin of the embryo. Muscles of the body are forming. Although the external genitals are still not distinct, ovaries and testes can be seen.

Accurate measurements of the growing embryo can be made by ultrasound. These measurements correlate very accurately

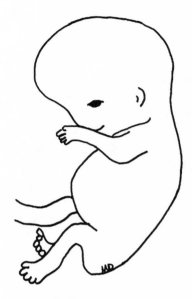

EIGHT-WEEK-OLD FETUS

with the age of the embryo at this stage. One measurement, called a crown-rump length, is taken from the top of the embryo's head to the bottom of its rump.

COMPLICATIONS THAT CAN OCCUR

Miscarriage and Ectopic Pregnancy

Both of these complications were discussed in the previous chapter.

WHEN TO CALL YOUR DOCTOR

Contact your doctor if you are experiencing any amount of bleeding, severe cramping, increasing lower abdominal pain or sudden severe abdominal pain. Also contact your health care provider if you are having unrelenting vomiting or diarrhea.

QUESTIONS

1. *Should I wear flat shoes now that I'm pregnant?*
   You won't need to wear flat shoes this early in pregnancy, but you should wear shoes that have a lower heel. Spike heels will throw you off balance as your pregnancy progresses.

2. *Can I sunbathe while I am pregnant?*

   Yes, there is no reason not to sunbathe as long as you use a good sunscreen and avoid the peak hours of the day. Keep yourself well hydrated when out in the sun. You also may want to follow your outing with a liberal application of skin moisturizer.

3. *Why don't I have morning sickness?*

   Some women are more sensitive to hormonal changes than others. If you don't experience morning sickness, that doesn't mean there's a problem with your pregnancy. It simply means you're lucky.

4. *Why do I cry at stupid fast-food commercials?*

   You may find that you have inappropriate responses to many situations while you're pregnant. This goes with the territory. Your emotions are very sensitive now. Accept that and you'll feel better.

CHAPTER SEVEN

I CAN'T BUTTON MY JEANS

Third Lunar Month of
Pregnancy

PHYSICAL CHANGES

Morning sickness should lessen by the twelfth week. Headaches and dizziness may have started. Constipation, heartburn, frequent urination and fatigue may all be present. You may notice more nasal congestion and nosebleeds. Increase in the maternal blood volume, thinning of mucus membranes in the nose and increased respiration can contribute to nasal congestion and nosebleeds. You may notice an increase in gassiness. Your clothes may be extremely tight or not fit anymore.

PEARL HARBOR DAY

Caitlin had spotting when she was eight weeks pregnant, but this had stopped and she was doing well. I had just left my office when my service paged me for an emergency. Gregory, Caitlin's husband, had called and said he must speak to me immediately. There was something wrong with his wife. I called, expecting to hear that she was bleeding again. However, that was not the case. Gregory told me that his wife had locked herself in the bedroom and was crying and would not come out. He was finally able to convince her to talk to me. Caitlin was very upset. They were going out and she had put on everything in her closet, but nothing fit. Clothes were not just tight, they could not be zipped. She had even tried lying down on her bed to zip her jeans. She had only gained two pounds; how could her clothes not fit? Something had to be wrong. I explained that her body was changing very rapidly and it was not dependent on the amount of weight she gained. Some women need loose maternity clothes sooner than others. Caitlin was not happy to be one of those women, but she was happy that nothing was wrong. She then pointed out that at least the day was appropriate. It was the anniversary of Pearl Harbor, and for her this would be a day she would never forget.

EMOTIONAL CHANGES

Mom

You may experience a growing or lessening interest in sex. Your mood swings may become more pronounced, and you may become more depressed as your body changes. You may spend more time on your hair and makeup to try to draw attention away from your body. You become more aware of how your clothes no longer fit. If you think you're becoming unattractive to your partner, you need to talk to him and let him know your fears.

Dad

You may become more frightened as mom's mood swings become more pronounced. She may seem more interested in her appearance and the pregnancy than in you. These are normal feelings. You need to talk to each other about your feelings. You may also find it helpful to talk to other pregnant fathers to compare notes. There are resources available for the expectant father (see appendices), and you may find them helpful.

YOUR PRENATAL VISIT

You should be seen four weeks after your last visit.

What Should Be Done

Weight

Blood pressure

Urinalysis for protein and glucose

Monitoring of fetal heartbeat (this is usually heard by the twelfth or thirteenth week using a Doppler)

Evaluation of the size of the uterus (it should be at the top of the pelvic bone by the twelfth week)

Examination of hands and feet for signs of swelling and varicose veins

Discussion of any problems or questions you both may have

Tests That May Be Done

CHORIONIC VILLUS SAMPLING (CVS)
CVS, performed between the ninth and eleventh week of pregnancy, is a test for chromosomal abnormalities. A small amount of placental tissue is removed from the uterus, using a thin catheter placed through the cervix with ultrasound guidance. The tissue is then grown in a culture. The cells are examined for abnormal chromosomes, both in the number and for certain enzymes. Cervical cultures for gonorrhea and chlamydia will be done before CVS is performed. It takes about two weeks to obtain results from a CVS. You may be a candidate for CVS if you have had a child with Down's syndrome; will be thirty-five at the time of delivery; or if you or your partner is a carrier of genetic abnormalities, such as Tay-Sachs disease, hemophilia and lethal enzyme deficiencies. The advantage of CVS is that it is performed

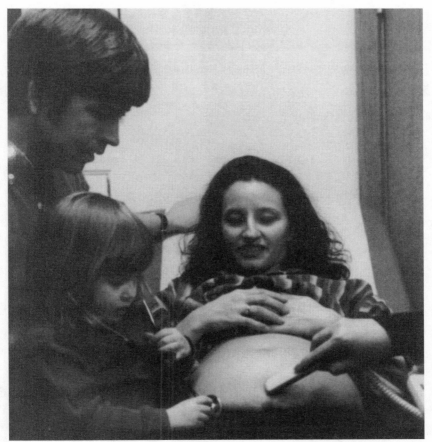

Bringing older children to prenatal visits makes them a part of the pregnancy.

very early in the pregnancy. If a major genetic abnormality is detected, the pregnancy can be safely terminated, if you desire that option. CVS carries a 3 to 5 percent risk of miscarriage. There have been reports of limb abnormalities in babies whose mothers have had a CVS done. However, you and your doctor should decide if the risks outweigh the benefits of this procedure. CVS should be performed by a highly trained specialist in maternal-fetal medicine.

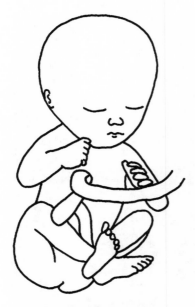

TWELVE-WEEK-OLD FETUS

WHAT YOU SHOULD BE DOING

You should decide how much you want to spend on maternity clothes and what type of clothes you want (see appendices). Leggings with oversize T-shirts or sweaters are a comfortable, non-pregnant look. Billowy dresses may also be appropriate for you. The traditional "maternity look" is not your only option today. You need to decide what is comfortable for you. After all, you'll be wearing these clothes for the next seven months.

Continue exercising; it's good for your body and self-esteem. Avoid gas-producing foods, such as cabbage, broccoli and beans.

If you haven't told your other children about the baby, it's time to begin preparing them. There are many books and tapes available to help you with this (see appendices). Bring the children with you to your prenatal visits. Talk about the new baby and when it will come. Always reassure the children that the new baby will never take their place and that you and Dad have enough love for everyone. Begin to discuss their role as a big brother or sister.

YOUR BABY

The fetal period begins with the ninth week of pregnancy. At ten weeks, the inch-and-a-half-long fetus is surrounded by fluid. It becomes more active and is able to move its tiny arms and legs. The yolk sac has begun to decrease in size as the fetal liver, spleen and bones take over its function. The baby's eyes are completely formed, and by the end of the twelfth week the eyelids have fused over the eyes. Sucking movements of the mouth can be seen, and the baby is noted to turn its head. The face has taken on a more humanlike quality. The tiny brain has begun to transmit messages to the fully formed, maturing body. The risk of miscarriage has decreased substantially by the end of this period.

COMPLICATIONS THAT CAN OCCUR

Late First-Trimester Miscarriage

Most first-trimester miscarriages will take place by the ninth week; however, they can occur up to the twelfth week. See pages 85–86 for a discussion on miscarriages.

Ectopic Pregnancy

See page 84 for a discussion.

WHEN TO CALL YOUR DOCTOR

Contact your doctor if you experience any bleeding, severe cramping or abdominal pain.

QUESTIONS

1. *What are early prenatal classes and should I attend?*
   If the hospital or birthing center you have chosen offers early prenatal classes, you may want to take them. They may give you details about nutrition, development of your baby and exercises and offer you the opportunity to interact with other couples who are pregnant.

2. *Should I wear seat belts now that I am getting bigger?*

   Absolutely. Seat belts save lives. The shoulder strap should be above your growing belly, the seat strap should be across your legs, not your growing uterus. By placing the belts in this manner, the fetus is protected from sudden trauma should you be in an accident.

CHAPTER EIGHT

MUSIC BOXES AND BEDTIME STORIES

Fourth Lunar Month of Pregnancy

PHYSICAL CHANGES

You will begin to notice a decrease in urinary frequency and the end of morning sickness. In fact, you may even experience an increase in appetite. You could be hungry all the time. You will have a great deal more energy by the end of this month. There will be a gradual increase in the amount of vaginal discharge you have. Although your breasts will continue to increase in size, they may become much less tender. You may notice a slight shortness of breath. Your heart rate will be faster and you may notice palpitations, a racing of your heart. This is normal if it occurs occasionally, but you should let your doctor know if it occurs. You may begin to "show" or have a bulging lower abdomen by the end of the fourth month. Sex is usually better because the vagina is more engorged with blood, making the thrusting more intense for most women. Some women experience orgasm or multiple orgasms for the first time during this period.

EMOTIONAL CHANGES

Mom

Your ability to concentrate may be challenged. The lack of concentration, of being "scatterbrained," is disturbing to most women. It's normal, though, as you spend more time thinking about your baby. You may also begin to feel that you are "fat" because you don't really look pregnant. Your mood swings can reflect this. The mood swings continue throughout the pregnancy, but your partner and others around you may have become used to them. It's time to become actively involved with your baby and to share this with your partner.

Dad

The pregnancy may still not be real for you. Your partner's body may not have changed dramatically and you can't feel the baby move yet. You've heard the heartbeat, but it somehow doesn't seem connected to what is happening to your partner. You should begin to talk to the baby during this time; you'll be surprised at how much closer you become to the baby and your partner.

YOUR PRENATAL VISIT

You should be seen four weeks after your last visit.

What Should Be Done

Weight

Blood pressure

Urinalysis for protein and glucose

Monitoring of fetal heartbeat

Measurement of the height of the fundus (the top of the uterus)

Evaluation of the size and shape of the uterus

Examination of hands and feet for swelling and varicose veins

Discussion of any problems or questions you both may have

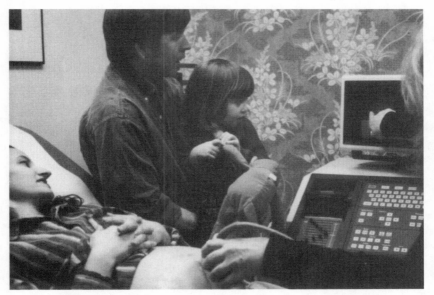

Mom, Dad and Big Sister-to-be watch the baby suck its thumb.

Tests That May Be Done

SONOGRAM

A sonogram, or ultrasound scan, uses sound waves to produce echoes of objects in water. These echoes are converted, by computer, to moving pictures on a screen. Ultrasound is not ionizing radiation and poses no risk to mom or the baby.

You will be asked to maintain a full bladder for this scan to allow the uterus to be pushed upward out of the pelvis. Your abdomen is covered with a water-soluble gel because sound waves travel through liquid. A probe is then placed on your abdomen and a moving picture of your baby is seen on the screen. You may even see your baby sucking its thumb.

Sonograms are done at various times during a pregnancy. They are used to identify any anatomic or developmental abnormalities; to check the size of the baby; to assist in such procedures as amniocentesis, CVS, fetoscopy (a procedure that examines the fetus directly in-utero through a special instrument) and fetal surgery; to confirm the baby's position near birth; to locate the placenta; to detect the number of babies present; and to assess how well the baby is doing.

In some countries, sonograms are performed twice during pregnancy, once at sixteen to eighteen weeks to assess fetal abnormalities, and again at thirty-two to thirty-four weeks to assess age and well-being. There is some controversy in this country on the need for sonograms in a normal pregnancy. However, I advise patients to have a sonogram at sixteen to eighteen weeks to assess fetal abnormalities.

ALPHA-FETOPROTEIN

Alpha-fetoprotein is produced by the fetal liver and is excreted through the placenta into the mother's blood. The mother is given a blood test, usually taken between fifteen and seventeen weeks, to determine the amount of alpha-fetoprotein present. A high amount could indicate that the baby has a neural tube defect, such as spina bifida (open spine) or anencephaly (absence of the brain). The incidence of spina bifida is 1 or 2 per 1,000. If you have had one child with spina bifida, your risk is 5 percent. The test can be positive 5 percent of the time, which means that further investigation is needed.

If the value of the alpha-fetoprotein test is high, the first step is to repeat it. A sonogram to determine the accurate fetal age is done, since values are dependent on the age of the fetus. If the second value is high, a high-resolution scan is done to look for neural tube defects. An amniocentesis may also be done to ascertain the exact amount of the substance in the amniotic fluid. If a defect is found, parents must make a decision on continuing the pregnancy based on the severity of the defect.

A low value could be indicative of Down's syndrome (a genetic condition that may include mental retardation and physical defects caused by an abnormal chromosomal number). An amniocentesis will be done to determine if the baby does have any genetic abnormality.

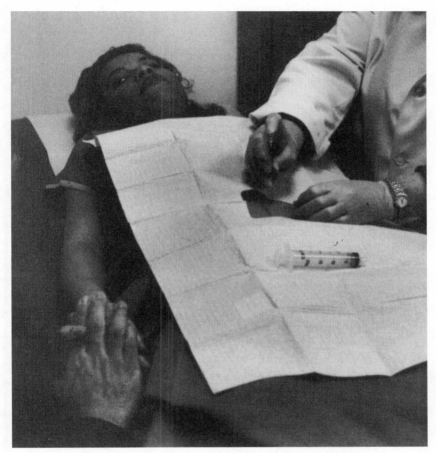

Having Dad present during the amniocentesis may calm both of you.

AMNIOCENTESIS

An amniocentesis, usually performed during the fourteenth to seventeenth week, is a test that analyzes the baby's amniotic fluid. Your abdomen is cleansed with a bacteriostatic solution and then, with ultrasound guidance, a thin needle in inserted and approximately 30 cubic centimeters of fluid is removed. The fluid is sent to a laboratory, where it is centrifuged. The cells from the fetus are separated from the fluid and cultured, or grown, in a special medium. It takes approximately eight days to three weeks to grow the cells. The cells are then analyzed for chromosomal abnormalities, such as Down's syndrome. The cells and fluid are also analyzed for enzyme defects found in such inherited diseases as Tay-Sachs and thalassemia. The sex of the baby is determined, since it is important to screen for such sex-linked diseases as hemophilia.

Couples at risk of having a child with genetic abnormalities should have an amniocentesis done. The risk of Down's syndrome increases with age. At a maternal age of twenty-seven, the risk is 1 per 1,000. At thirty-five, the risk increases to 1 per 400; at forty, 1 per 100; and at forty-five, 1 per 30. There is evidence that the risk of Down's syndrome increases for fathers over the age of fifty.

Amniocentesis is also used to evaluate the amniotic fluid bilirubin, a substance found when red blood cells are destroyed, in Rh-sensitized babies. Later in pregnancy, amniocentesis can evaluate fetal lung maturity by measuring two substances, lecithin and sphingomyelin, and looking at the ratio of one to the other. Fetal oxygenation can also be assessed using amniocentesis.

The risk factor of amniocentesis is about 0.5 percent. The risks include possible infection, miscarriage and loss of amniotic fluid. You will need to discuss both the risks and benefits with your doctor.

Postamniocentesis Instructions

1. After the test, you should go home, put your feet up and take it easy for the rest of the day.

2. Mild cramping for a short time is to be expected. If the cramping becomes severe or does not dissipate in several hours, call your doctor's office.

3. The most common complication of amniocentesis is leaking of amniotic fluid. If you notice a clear watery discharge within the following twenty-four hours, call the office immediately.

4. Over several days following the test, fever greater than 100 degrees, abdominal pain or vaginal bleeding should be reported immediately.

5. By the following day you should be perfectly able to perform your usual activities.

6. The difficult part has just begun—the waiting. It takes from eight days to three and a half weeks for results. The time varies and is not indicative of a problem with your pregnancy. The cells found in the amniotic fluid are allowed to divide in a culture medium. Some methods take longer than others.

7. If you have any questions, contact your doctor. Even if you think the questions may be silly or unimportant, he or she will want to hear from you.

WHAT YOU SHOULD BE DOING

Several years ago, I embarked on a study to find a way for mom and dad to get in touch with their unborn child. Using medical facts gleaned about children of the Holocaust, a study of Eastern cultures and research in developmental embryology, I developed my "Music Boxes and Bedtime Stories" method of fetal conditioning. Research has established that babies can recognize the voices of their fathers as well as their mothers. Using fetal conditioning, both mom and dad can bond with the baby before birth and establish a family unit.

To include this method in your pregnancy, first choose a music box song that you both like; after all, you will be living with it for at least a year. I suggest, though, that you not tell anyone what your song is (the following anecdote will illustrate why).

DON'T PLAY IT AGAIN, SAM

My daughter followed my theories while my grandson, Samuel, was ges-tating. The song she chose was "Somewhere Over the Rainbow." She was very excited that the baby seemed to "listen" to the music nightly and would become very active when she played the music box on her stomach. After playing, she would talk quietly to the baby and soothe him. When Samuel was born, he recognized the song immediately. If crying, he would stop and listen. He also would fall asleep to it. Since everyone thought this was wonderful, my daughter received forty-three baby gifts, each one playing "Somewhere Over the Rainbow." If I never hear the song again, I will be a happy woman. Samuel still tells everyone that it was his baby song; however, only Dorothy of Kansas is allowed to sing it now.

You and your partner next need to establish a consistent, daily, quiet moment together. This will be your "family time." You will find that you continue this practice after the baby is born. If you have older children, they should be allowed to participate in this period and talk to the baby.

You should both relax and get in touch with each other, discuss the problems of the day and your feelings about the pregnancy. Dad needs to talk to the baby directly. Since some men feel self-conscious about doing this, I suggest you read to your baby. The choice of reading material is yours. I have had fathers who read the baseball scores, stock quotes and children's books, such as *The Velveteen Rabbit*. What you read and say is not as important as the tone of your voice and the repetition of doing this every day for at least a half hour.

After dad has finished reading, place the music box on your stomach and play it for about ten to fifteen minutes. The baby will usually react to this with a flurry of activity. This accomplishes two things. First, it gets the baby used to, or conditioned to, the song. Second, the activity causes an increase in heart rate, which increases bloodflow to the developing brain.

Follow the music period by talking quietly to the baby in a reassuring voice. This can also be a good time for you to begin practicing meditation techniques that can relieve stress and be used in labor. By repeating this activity on a daily basis, you are establishing quiet family time and conditioning your baby to the sound of your voices in a calm atmosphere. If you follow this regimen,

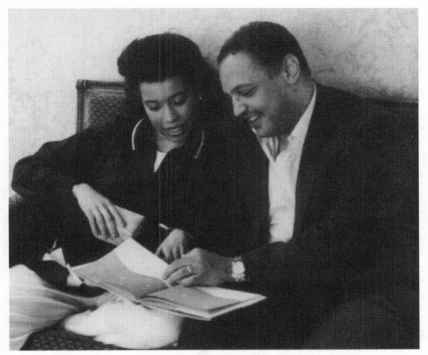

*Fetal conditioning gives Mom and Dad quiet time together and
helps Dad begin to bond with the baby.*

when your baby is born it will react to both parents' voices, be
awake and alert and can be calmed to the sounds of its music box
song.

We know that maternal stress can cause problems for the baby.
Constant stress situations can result in babies who do not grow
well. Meditation and visualization are excellent ways to relieve
stress and anxiety and produce a calm atmosphere for you and
your baby. Your baby reacts with you to situations. Using the techniques described earlier in this book is an excellent way to learn
meditation. You can also use these technique to help you deal
with labor. Beginning the daily practice of meditation now not
only will provide a release for your stress but will make meditation
a very natural technique to use in labor.

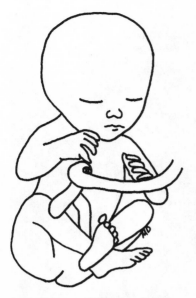

SIXTEEN-WEEK-OLD FETUS

YOUR BABY

By the end of this period, all organ systems are completely functional. The external genitalia have formed and are recognizable. The senses are developing; the baby now can taste, hear and react to sound. Eyebrows and eyelashes are beginning and the baby can smile, frown, even suck its thumb. The hands can form fists and grasp.

COMPLICATIONS THAT CAN OCCUR

This is a time when problems with the fetus are discovered. Fetal surgery, a highly specialized area of medicine, is able to correct some of these problems. However, it is limited to a few routine procedures. Intrauterine blood transfusions are done under ultrasound guidance for Rh-sensitized babies. If hydronephrosis (swelling of the ureters, the tubes from the kidneys to the bladder) is discovered, a small plastic tube can be placed in the bladder to avoid permanent kidney damage to the baby.

Operating on the fetus outside the uterus is done rarely and only in highly specialized centers. This carries a tremendous risk to the baby and is done only for conditions that are life-threatening if allowed to continue. The mother is given general anesthesia; thus, the fetus also receives general anesthesia. The mother's abdomen is opened, then the uterus and membranes surrounding the fetus are opened. The amniotic fluid is drained and kept warm. The fetus is removed from the uterus and the necessary surgery performed. The baby is then placed back into the membranes, the membranes are closed and the fluid is replaced. The uterus and abdomen are then closed. The mother is placed on medication to prevent infection and the onset of early labor. When the baby is old enough to be born, it is delivered by c-section.

QUESTIONS

1. How many sonograms are safe to have?

No risk has been found for the baby. If you're worried about the number of sonograms, ask your doctor not to perform one before ten weeks and to limit the number later in pregnancy.

2. Will alpha-fetoprotein tests determine all cases of Down's syndrome?

No. The test can determine only about 20 percent of cases. A newer test, evaluating two other enzymes or hormones as well as alpha-fetoprotein, has a better detection rate; it can determine up to 70 percent of Down's syndrome cases. However, this test is not widely available.

3. Should I have an amniocentesis if I'm not prepared to terminate the pregnancy?

Yes, you may need to make preparations for the delivery. Some genetic problems have physical problems associated with them. You may therefore need to have specialists present at the delivery. You may also want to contact support groups for special needs children (see appendices).

✵ CHAPTER NINE

BUTTERFLIES GALORE

Fifth Lunar Month of
Pregnancy

PHYSICAL CHANGES

The baby is moving! You feel flutters at first, although not every day. You may also experience pain in the lower abdomen. These are round ligament pains caused by stretching of the ligaments on either side of the uterus. Your heart rate has increased due to an increase in blood volume and the need to get oxygen to the growing baby. You may begin to notice color changes in your skin. Mild swelling of your feet and ankles at the end of the day is not unusual, especially in hot weather. Your abdomen is growing and you look pregnant.

EMOTIONAL CHANGES

Mom

The reality of your pregnancy has finally set in with the baby's movements. You'll notice less mood swings now; however, you may still be irritable. The absentmindedness will continue and is normal. You'll think more about what your baby will be like. You may feel closer to your partner now. This will definitely be true if you have been practicing your nightly family time.

Dad

The reality of parenthood has set in. The baby is real and it moves. For some men, this is an exciting time during the pregnancy. However, as excited as you are, you may also feel frightened. These are normal feelings and you should discuss them with your partner. Use family time to discuss these thoughts.

YOUR PRENATAL VISIT

You should be seen four weeks after your last visit.

What Should Be Done

Weight

Blood pressure

Urinalysis for protein and glucose

Monitoring of fetal heartbeat

Measurement of the height of the fundus

Evaluation of the size and shape of the uterus

Examination of hands and feet for signs of swelling and varicose veins

Discussion of any problems or questions you both may have

WHAT YOU SHOULD BE DOING

You should continue your quiet family time every day.

Since you may be hungry more often, you should eat nutritious snacks, such as yogurt, rather than empty calories, as found in cookies and candy. Your exercise regimen should continue.

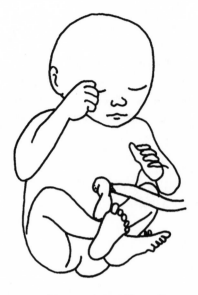

TWENTY-WEEK-OLD FETUS

Travel should be more comfortable now, but remember to avoid sitting in one position too long. Your clothing should be loose and comfortable.

YOUR BABY

Your nine- to ten-inch-long baby now has fully formed ears and growing fingernails. It feels touch and reacts to it. Fingerprints have formed. The baby is covered with fine hair called lanugo, over which is a cheeselike covering called vernix. It now actively sucks its thumb and swallows, and breathes the amniotic fluid to help the growing lungs expand.

COMPLICATIONS THAT CAN OCCUR

Premature Cervical Dilation

Premature cervical dilation is a rare condition in which the cervix opens before the due date. The incompetent cervix can result from previous surgery, such as cone biopsy, and tears of the cervix in an earlier delivery. It can also be a spontaneous condition. There is no warning that this will happen. No labor precedes it. The cervix opens and the fetus is expelled. If the condition is found in time, a stitch can be placed in the cervix to close it. Using a heavy, nonabsorbable suture material, a purse-string stitch called a cerclage is placed and pulled to close the opening in the cervix. A second stitch may be placed. When premature cervical dilation occurs during this time in the pregnancy, there is a 50 percent chance that the pregnancy will continue. There is a high rate of infection, because the membranes around the baby have been exposed to the bacteria in the vagina. The stitch is cut and removed about two weeks before the due date, and usually a vaginal delivery is possible.

This condition usually occurs at the same time in every pregnancy. If you have a history of an incompetent cervix, the stitch can be placed at thirteen weeks of pregnancy. This will allow the pregnancy to continue until term.

WHEN TO CALL YOUR DOCTOR

Contact your doctor if you notice a pink or blood-tinged discharge—this may indicate cervical dilation. Also, contact him or her if you have a sudden gush of fluid, contractions or pressure in the vagina.

STANDING ON MY HEAD

Carla called me to report a fullness in her vagina when she awakened one day during her nineteenth week of pregnancy. I met her and her husband at the hospital, where I discovered that her cervix had dilated to four centimeters and the membranes were bulging into the vagina. She was placed in a bed that tilted her body head down. A tocolytic, a medication that stops premature labor, was begun. The operating room was prepared for Carla. The membranes were pushed back into the uterus and a cerclage was placed in her cervix. She was taken back to the labor floor, where she was kept in a head-down position for twenty-four hours, still receiving tocolytics. She was also placed on antibiotics to prevent infection. After twenty-four hours, she was allowed to sit up in bed, then to get out of bed. No labor occurred and Carla was sent home on bedrest. The stitch was removed in the office at thirty-eight weeks of pregnancy. I received a call that night that Carla was in labor.

We went to the hospital and she gave birth to a wonderful, healthy daughter.

QUESTIONS

---

1. ***Does round ligament pain hurt my baby?***

   No, round ligament pain only bothers you. The baby doesn't notice it.

CHAPTER TEN

THE ALL-NIGHT DANCE PARTIES

Sixth Lunar Month of Pregnancy

PHYSICAL CHANGES

The activity of your baby has increased greatly. It still varies from day to day, but the baby has stronger kicks and increased movement. The round ligament pain should be gone by the end of this month. You may begin to notice leg cramps, especially at night. Your abdomen may begin to itch as your skin stretches to accommodate the growing uterus. Stretch marks may have started. Backaches are common from now on in pregnancy, as are hemorrhoids. You may notice that your feet swell by the end of the day. Your appetite is good. Traveling, with precautions, is not a problem. Sex is still comfortable.

UP ALL NIGHT

Jean Anne and Colin were very excited about feeling the baby move. At her twenty-week visit, she said she couldn't wait until the baby moved all the time. But when Jean Anne came in for her 24-week visit, she had a different point of view. She was now as tired as she had been at the beginning of her pregnancy and told me that she hadn't been able to get more than two or three hours of sleep a night. The baby was up all night and was extremely active. Upon questioning, she said that she had consumed caffeine during the late afternoon. She also said the baby slept all day when she was at work. I suggested that she discontinue caffeine use after three in the afternoon and try meditation before going to bed.

I also suggested that she try to rearrange her work schedule so that her busy and stressful time was earlier in the day. Jean Anne called about a week later and said that she was now getting four or five hours of sleep a night, as well as a nap in the morning. The baby still liked nighttime activity, but he had settled down enough for his mother to get some sleep.

EMOTIONAL CHANGES

Mom

You will begin to focus more on your baby. You may begin to obsess on whether your baby will be all right. Everything you do may cause you to think of the effects on the baby. Stress levels are higher now as the pregnancy advances. Discuss your feelings with your partner.

Dad

You become more aware of the baby and its safety now. The baby is moving and you can feel it. You worry about what kind of father you will be and how you will handle the responsibility of parenthood. You may be distressed because your partner is turning inward. These are all normal emotions and you should discuss them with your partner. She's having the same feelings.

YOUR PRENATAL VISIT

You should be seen four weeks after your last visit.

What Should Be Done

Weight

Blood pressure

Urinalysis for protein and glucose

Monitoring of fetal heartbeat

Measurement of the height of the fundus

Evaluation of the size and shape of the uterus

Examination of hands and feet for signs of swelling and varicose veins

Discussion of any problems or questions you both may have

WHAT YOU SHOULD BE DOING

Leg cramps may be caused by a decrease in your calcium level. Before bedtime try taking an antacid that contains calcium. If this doesn't alleviate the cramping, your doctor may prescribe calcium supplements. Swelling of the feet is common, and you should keep your feet elevated as much as possible during the day. Backaches can be soothed by massages administered by your partner or a masseuse who knows maternal massage techniques. Wearing low-heeled or flat shoes will also keep backaches to a minimum. If you are active all day, a belly bra may help alleviate your backaches. This is a slinglike garment that can be found at maternity shops.

Eating a high-fiber diet and drinking plenty of fluids will keep your stool soft, and thus the pain and bleeding of hemorrhoids will be kept to a minimum. If hemorrhoids continue to bother you, ask your doctor for a stool softener and medication to help shrink the hemorrhoids.

Liberally apply moisturizers that contain lanolin or cocoa butter and aloe to your skin. This will alleviate the itching, which is caused by the stretching of the fibers in your skin.

Continue to have your family time and to meditate. Meditation helps to relieve stress. This period is also an ideal time for you and your partner to discuss and prepare for the emotional

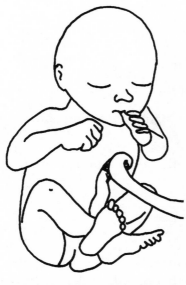

TWENTY-FOUR-WEEK-OLD FETUS

changes that parenthood will bring to your relationship.

Now is the time to make reservations for prepared childbirth classes.

YOUR BABY

Your baby's skin has become more opaque, red and wrinkled. The baby has established a sleep-wake pattern. Tiny teeth buds have begun to develop. The lungs are completely formed; however, it will still be twelve weeks before the baby can breathe air without problems.

COMPLICATIONS THAT CAN OCCUR

Although bladder infections are not really complications of pregnancy, they can lead to other problems, such as premature labor, if they're not treated. Your doctor will check your urine at each visit for protein. A positive reading may indicate a bladder infection. Urinary tract infections are common during pregnancy and are easily treated with oral antibiotics.

Another common problem in pregnancy is a yeast infection. The increased production of glucose to feed the growing baby changes the environment of the vagina, allowing yeast to grow more easily.

WHEN TO CALL YOUR DOCTOR

Contact your doctor if you notice pain upon urination, increased frequency of urination or lower abdominal pain—these can signal a urinary tract infection. Also contact him or her if you notice vaginal odor, a change in color of your discharge or vaginal itchiness.

QUESTIONS

1. *What causes a "pins and needles" sensation in my hand?*

   The sensation comes from a condition called carpal tunnel syndrome. As your body adds extra fluid, the tissues swell. The tissues of the wrists are protected by a fibrous band called a retinaculum, which does not expand. The median nerve, which goes to your thumb and middle two fingers, is within this fibrous band. As the tissues swell, the nerve is pressed; this results in the carpal tunnel syndrome. The condition may be helped by elevating your hands on a pillow and by wearing simple splints, even bowling gloves, at night. This condition usually goes away after pregnancy.

2. *How can I prevent stretch marks?*

   You can't. Save your money on those lotions and creams that promise to make your stretch marks disappear or that claim to prevent them. Elastic fibers in the skin are broken when the skin stretches to accommodate the growing baby. These will fade to a faint silvery color after pregnancy.

3. I have a dark line that runs between my belly button and pubic hair. What is it?

The line is called the linea nigra and results from the increased amounts of melanocyte-stimulating hormone that is present in pregnancy. Like all skin and pigmentation changes that occur in pregnancy, it will fade after the baby is born.

CHAPTER ELEVEN

FINDING YOUR DOCTOR SPOCK

Seventh Lunar Month of
Pregnancy

PHYSICAL CHANGES

The baby is kicking more vigorously, and this may be visible to the outside world. The baby will also begin to hiccup. You will notice an increased swelling of the feet and ankles at the end of the day, especially in the summer. You will gradually become short of breath more easily as the pregnancy progresses. Your body temperature is elevated over nonpregnant levels, so you are warm most of the time. Sleeping may now have become a real problem as your insomnia increases. You may be thrown off balance and be clumsier as the pregnancy progresses. The uterus has begun to practice for labor, and you will notice that you have contractions occasionally. These are called Braxton-Hicks contractions. They are irregular and of varying intensity.

OH MY GOD, IT'S MOVING AGAIN

Serena, who was twenty-five weeks pregnant, became very stressed before giving presentations at work. During her reports, everyone would stop looking at the blackboard and stare at her stomach in amazement. The baby felt the stress she was under and reacted by kicking hard enough to be visible. During her prenatal visit after one such episode, Serena requested a prescription for an "Executive Baby Tranquilizer."

EMOTIONAL CHANGES

Mom

You may notice that you're more absentminded and fantasize more about the baby, now that he or she is moving all the time. You also may be having renewed fears about the baby's well-being. Can you be a good mother, wife and career woman all at the same time? All of these thoughts may be racing through your head.

Dad

You'll probably feel closer to the baby, more connected, now. As you notice the baby's movements more often, you'll feel that the child knows you. This will be more evident if the baby moves to the sound of your voice.

I'M THE ONLY ONE THIS BABY KNOWS

Jason was a very zealous dad. He even called his wife during the day and asked her to put the phone to her stomach so that he could talk to the baby. He was absolutely convinced that his baby responded only to his voice. In fact, he even called the baby Igor and said the baby responded to his name. During the prenatal visits, Jason would talk to the baby, and indeed there was an increase in activity and heart rate.

YOUR PRENATAL VISIT

You should be seen four weeks after your last visit.

What Should Be Done

Weight

Blood pressure

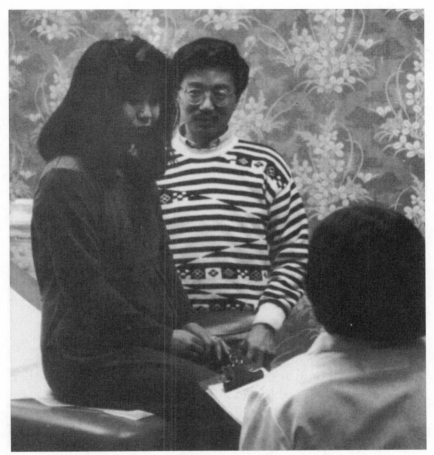

Don't forget to write down your questions and take them to your visit.

Urinalysis for protein and glucose

Measurement of the height of the fundus

Evaluation of the size and shape of the uterus

Examination of hands and feet for signs of swelling and varicose veins

Discussion of any problems or questions you both may have

Tests That May Be Done

GLUCOSE TEST

A glucose test screens for gestational diabetes. You will be given a sugar-water drink that contains 50 grams of glucose. An hour later, blood will be drawn to measure the amount of glucose present in your blood. If your value is higher than 130 mg/dl, you will be scheduled for a three-hour glucose tolerance test in which a fasting blood glucose level is obtained. You will then drink 100 grams of sugar water. Blood will be taken thirty minutes, one hour, two hours and three hours later. Abnormal values indicate gestational diabetes.

BLOOD TEST FOR RH ANTIBODIES IN RH NEGATIVE MOTHERS

If you are Rh negative, blood will be drawn to determine if you have developed antibodies to Rh positive blood.

WHAT YOU SHOULD BE DOING

Now is the best time to begin putting the baby's nursery together. You're more comfortable and able to move more easily than you will be in later pregnancy. Shopping for baby furniture can be fun, but have an idea of what you want before you start your expedition. (A list of nursery and layette items can be found in the appendices.) There's no reason you can't be around when the baby's room is being painted or wallpapered; latex paint won't harm you or your baby. However, you should make sure the area is well ventilated.

It's also time to find your Dr. Spock. Your baby's pediatrician will be a very important person in all your lives for the next several years. But you shouldn't make any decision without doing some legwork. Conduct interviews. Decide if you'll like this doctor. Will he or she be responsive to your calls? How does he or she handle emergencies? These are only a few of the questions you should have. (A more complete list of interview questions can be

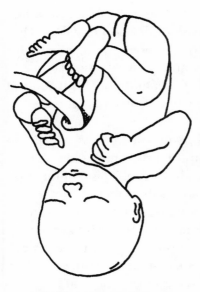

TWENTY-EIGHT-WEEK-OLD FETUS

found in the appendices.) If a pediatrician doesn't have time to see you now, perhaps he or she won't have time when you really need help later.

Finding your Dr. Spock may not be as difficult as you think. Ask friends and coworkers for suggestions. Ask your doctor for a recommendation. Hospitals also maintain a registry of doctors on their staff and may be able to recommend several to you. You should interview several pediatricians before you choose.

YOUR BABY

Your baby opens and closes its eyes and can taste, smell and see light. The baby's skin is thicker and its body temperature is self-regulated. The urinary tract can now produce urine.

COMPLICATIONS THAT CAN OCCUR

Gestational Diabetes Mellitus

About 3 percent of pregnant women will develop gestational diabetes. This will go away after the pregnancy ends; however, some studies have shown that up to 50 percent of gestational diabetics will develop diabetes later in life. Gestational diabetes mellitus (GDM) happens when your body cannot produce enough insulin to handle the increased glucose present in pregnancy. Women who are obese, have a family history of diabetes, have a previous baby that weighed more than nine pounds at birth, or have had a stillbirth may be at an increased risk of developing GDM. During pregnancy, women with gestational diabetes may experience an increase in frequency of bladder and yeast infections.

Glucose levels can be controlled by diet and possibly insulin. It is extremely important for your baby that your blood glucose levels be controlled.

A sustained, high glucose level in you will cause your baby to grow larger than it should. More importantly, a high glucose level can cause your baby to not get enough oxygen. This combination of hyperglycemia and hypoxemia can result in fetal death.

Babies of mothers with GDM are watched very carefully and are delivered as soon as their lungs are mature. You will have a complete sonogram every four weeks, a non-stress test twice a week and a biophysical profile once a week. An amniocentesis will be done at thirty-seven or thirty-eight weeks to test for fetal lung maturity. If the baby's lungs are mature, you will be delivered. Because babies of mothers with GDM may have trouble with calcium and glucose regulation, your baby will be taken to the neonatal intensive care nursery, where it will be monitored for twenty-four hours.

Premature (Preterm) Labor and Birth

Identifying premature labor is difficult. The current criteria are contractions occurring every four to five minutes that persist for more than one hour and last for thirty seconds. These contractions must cause dilation and effacement of the cervix in a pregnancy less than thirty-seven weeks gestation.

Premature labor can be caused by hypertension, uterine abnormalities such as fibroids and DES exposure, multiple babies, infections, cervical incompetence, placenta previa, premature rupture of membranes, preeclampsia, abruptio placentae and dehydration. However, 40 percent of the time no cause can be identified. Premature babies are less than 37 weeks gestation and weigh less than five-and-one half pounds.

Premature babies can have multiple problems, including respiratory distress, or difficulty breathing due to lung immaturity. Sometimes preterm labor should not be stopped, such as when ruptured membranes, abruptio placentae or infection is detected. However, if the baby and mother are healthy, attempts are made to stop labor. After all, mom is still the best incubator.

If you go into premature labor, you will be admitted to the hospital for complete bedrest and hydration with IV fluids. This stops contractions 50 percent of the time. If contractions do not stop, IV medications called tocolytics will be administered. Tocolytics, drugs that decrease or eliminate contractions, work only 30 to 40 percent of the time. Once contractions have stopped for at least twenty-four hours, you will be given tocolytics orally and the IVs will be stopped. You will then gradually be allowed limited walking, such as going to the bathroom. With the introduction of portable contraction monitoring devices, patients are now able to go home and stay in bed rather than be hospitalized.

If labor cannot be stopped, your baby will be delivered with extreme caution. During labor, the baby will be monitored continuously. An epidural will be administered. During delivery an episiotomy, a cut made to expand the opening of the vagina, will be done. This allows for less pressure and trauma to the baby's soft head. Forceps may also be used to protect the baby's head. A cesarean section may be done if your baby is very, very early.

Rh Iso-Immunization

Rh antigen is found in red blood cells and forms early in fetal life. However, 15 percent of white Americans and 5 percent of black Americans do not have this antigen. The antigen is a dominant genetic trait, which means that if one of the two genes that produce the antigen is positive and the other is negative, that individual will have the Rh antigen present and will be Rh positive. If

Rh positive blood is mixed with Rh negative blood, antibodies will form that will destroy blood cells that have the Rh antigen. This does not happen when Rh positive and Rh positive blood are mixed, nor when Rh negative and Rh negative are mixed.

If an Rh negative woman and an Rh positive man are pregnant, the possibility of a baby that has Rh positive blood is 60 percent. If a small amount of the baby's blood mixes with the mother's, the mother could make antibodies against the baby's blood. This is called Rh iso-immunization. If this occurs, the antibodies can be detected by a blood test. These antibodies can cross the placenta and destroy the baby's red blood cells.

RhoGAM, an Rh immunoglobulin, prevents the mother from forming antibodies. RhoGAM cannot be used if the mother already has antibodies.

If you are Rh negative, an antibody test will be done at twenty-eight weeks. If the test is negative, you will be given an injection of RhoGAM. You will also be given RhoGAM if you have had a CVS or amniocentesis. You will receive RhoGAM within seventy-two hours of delivery if your baby is Rh positive.

WHEN TO CALL YOUR DOCTOR

Contact your doctor if you experience a headache that is not relieved by acetaminophen, rest or meditation; if you are less than thirty-seven weeks pregnant and your membranes rupture; or if you are less than thirty-seven weeks pregnant and you experience contractions that last at least thirty seconds and occur every four or five minutes for at least one hour.

QUESTIONS

1. *Will tocolytics harm my baby?*
   There has been no long-term effects found in babies whose mothers received tocolytics.

2. I sometimes have a pain that runs down my back, buttock, and leg. What is it, and is there anything I can do for it?

This is sciatic nerve compression, which is caused by the weight of the baby and uterus on the sciatic nerve, which runs through the pelvis. To relieve the pain, get down on your hands and knees and lower your chest to the floor, resting your head on your arms. Stay in this position for a few moments, then get up slowly. This will shift the weight and position of the baby and uterus, temporarily providing relief.

CHAPTER TWELVE

WHAT HAPPENED TO MY FEET?

*Eighth Lunar Month of
Pregnancy*

PHYSICAL CHANGES

You will notice an increase in Braxton-Hicks contractions. Shortness of breath seems to be present with any exertion. All of your skin may seem itchy. Your breasts have stopped growing, but you may notice a thin, white, opaque discharge. This is colostrum, the substance you make to feed the baby before your milk comes.

EMOTIONAL CHANGES

Mom

You're getting attention from everyone now; even strangers will come up and talk to you. Enjoy it! After all, once the baby is born, you may feel like the forgotten woman. You may also be hearing horror stories and old wives' tales about delivery. All the advice and stories you are hearing are from well-meaning people. They mean no harm; take what they say with a grain of salt. If in doubt, ask your doctor. Remember, pregnant women are not always rational.

THE GREEN BABY

Diane, the director of nursing at a leading private hospital, called the office and asked to speak with me. She said it wasn't an emergency, but it was important. When I returned her call, she asked me to wait while she closed her office door. She seemed a bit hesitant and embarrassed about what she needed to ask me. Finally, she told me she had lunch in the cafeteria that day. One of the cafeteria workers, who noticed her daily diet, told her she was eating too much spinach. In fact, she had spinach every day. She told me she could never eat it before she got pregnant, but now she loved it. The worker then proceeded to inform her that if she continued to eat so much spinach her baby would be green-tinged when it was born. Of course, she knew this was ridiculous . . . but, she had been thinking about it. She decided she would call, even though it was silly, just to be sure. I assured her that her baby would not be green, just healthy from all the good food she was eating.

Perfectly intelligent, rational women will not always be that way while pregnant. Instead of worrying about things needlessly, call your doctor.

You will notice that you're even more absentminded now. You feel more stressed. These are all normal feelings. Share them with your partner.

Dad

You may be feeling left out as your partner is getting more and more attention now. Everyone seems to have forgotten you. You may begin to feel that you're not even necessary. Of course you are. Your partner needs your love and reassurance now more than ever, just as you need hers. Tell her.

You may also be having fears about the impending birth. Will you be able to handle it? What if you don't get to the hospital on time? These are normal thoughts. Express them.

YOUR PRENATAL VISITS

You will be seen two weeks after your last visit and every two weeks until the thirty-sixth week.

What Should Be Done

Weight

Blood pressure

Urinalysis for protein and glucose

Monitoring of fetal heartbeat

Measurement of the height of the fundus

Evaluation of the size and shape of the uterus

Examination of hands and feet for signs of swelling and varicose veins

Discussion of any problems or questions you both may have

Tests That May Be Done

If you have developed problems during your pregnancy or if you have a medical condition that could affect your pregnancy, your doctor will order tests that can assess how well your baby is doing.

BABY MOVEMENTS
Mom will be the first one to notice any difference in the baby's movements. No matter what your baby's activity pattern is, your baby should move at least ten times in two hours. The count should be made during the baby's usual activity time. For most babies, this is in the evening. A change in activity patterns should also be noted.

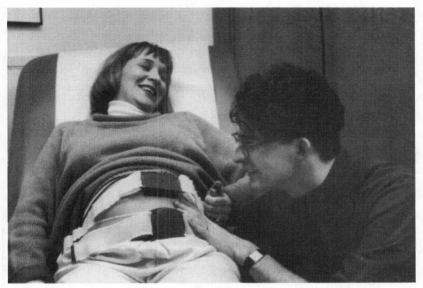

Sometimes Dad's voice will cause the baby to kick during a non-stress test.

NON-STRESS TEST (NST)

An NST measures the well-being of the baby based on the relationship between the baby's heart rate and activity. A monitor that transmits the baby's heartbeat is placed on you. Another monitor that detects uterine contractions is also hooked up. You then press a button every time the baby moves. The baby's heart rate should accelerate, by fifteen beats for at least fifteen seconds, twice in a twenty-minute period. This is called a reactive NST and is a good sign that the baby is healthy.

CONTRACTION STRESS TEST (CST)

If the baby does not have a reactive NST, your doctor may order a CST. A mild solution containing pitocin, a medication that causes contractions, is given intravenously. A fetal monitor is placed on the uterus. The amount of solution given is increased until contractions are recorded every three minutes. The effect of the contractions on the baby's heart rate is observed. There are three possible results. A reactive negative test shows accelerations of the baby's heart rate. With this result, the test may be repeated in one week. A nonreactive negative result is one in which no accelerations are seen, but no decelerations (a decrease in heart rate) are detected either. The test should be repeated in twenty-four hours if this result is obtained. A nonreactive positive test shows de-celerations related to the contractions. With this result, your doctor may do a biophysical profile or elect to deliver the baby. However, since there is a high rate of false positive results with this test, most doctors do a biophysical profile.

BIOPHYSICAL PROFILE (BPP)
Ultrasound has enabled doctors to assess babies' general health even before birth. Several parameters are observed:

1. *Breathing*—Does the baby have breathing movements at least once in thirty minutes?
2. *Body movement*—Does the baby move at least three times in thirty minutes?
3. *Muscle tone*—Does the baby have at least one flexion-extension (open-close) movement of arms, legs or hands in thirty minutes?
4. *NST*—Is it reactive?
5. *Amount of amniotic fluid*—Is there enough fluid around the baby?

Each of these is assigned a number. The numbers are then added to get a score: 8 to 10 is good, 6 is worrisome, 4 or below is ominous. Your doctor may decide to deliver your baby if the score is 6 or below.

WHAT YOU SHOULD BE DOING

Now is the time to start childbirth classes. You should be working on the baby's nursery and perhaps even finishing it. Of course, you are continuing family time.

It's also time to choose a name for the baby, if you haven't already done so. Choosing a name that you both like can be one of the most difficult things you have to do during this pregnancy. You and your partner may have different ideas of what the name should be. Just a few words of caution:

1. Your child will carry this name all its life.
2. Think about the picture you get of an adult with this name.
3. Say the entire name out loud to hear how it sounds.
4. Write the name.
5. Write the initials—do they spell anything? An example of this is Samuel Adam Peterson, a lovely name. The initials S A P, however, have another meaning.

Your older children can attend a sibling class this month. There they will see babies and learn what to expect.

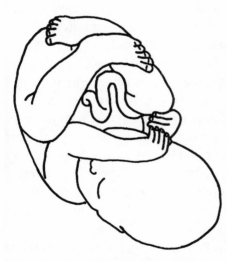

THIRTY-TWO-WEEK-OLD FETUS

YOUR BABY

By the time your baby is thirty-two weeks old, it has received your immunities from disease. The fetus can focus and blink its eyes. The lanugo has been shed, except over the back and shoulders, and real hair has started to grow. The baby has more body fat and weighs three to five pounds. It is beginning to run out of room and can't move as freely.

HOW MUCH ROOM IS THERE?

Karen's husband, Dan, a real estate developer, was very concerned about how much room the baby still had. At Karen's thirty-two-week visit, he seemed anxious to ask his questions. After I told them that everything seemed to be going well, Dan asked, "How much room does the baby have in there?" I told him the baby still had room to grow, but that answer didn't seem to satisfy him. He wanted more specific information. He asked, "Does the baby have as much room as an efficiency apartment or a two-bedroom condo?" I assured him that there would be adequate additions made to accommodate the baby's growth.

COMPLICATIONS THAT CAN OCCUR

Placenta Previa

Placenta previa means "placenta first." It is exactly what it sounds like. In this condition, the placenta has grown over the opening of the cervix. This occurs in about 1 in 200 pregnancies. The baby cannot be born vaginally with this condition.

The first sign of placenta previa may be bright red bleeding after sex. Any painless bright red bleeding at this point in pregnancy needs to be investigated. You will be admitted to the hospital and a sonogram will confirm the placenta's location. You will be kept on bedrest and watched. If bleeding occurs, you may be transfused if the blood loss is great enough. The baby will be observed closely for any signs of distress. If a major hemorrhage occurs, you will be delivered by emergency cesarean section. If no further bleeding occurs, an amniocentesis will be done at thirty-six or thirty-seven weeks to test for the baby's lung maturity. If the baby's lungs are mature, you will have a cesarean section delivery.

Premature Rupture of Membranes (PROM)

Premature rupture of membranes (PROM) is defined as ruptured membranes at least one hour before the onset of labor. Premature PROM occurs before thirty-seven weeks gestation. The cause of premature PROM is unknown, but infection may be involved 15 percent of the time.

Premature PROM, not accompanied by labor within an hour, is managed conservatively as long as signs of infection or fetal distress are not present. You are placed on bedrest and the baby is monitored closely. About 70 to 80 percent of women with premature PROM will go into labor within a week. After thirty-seven or thirty-eight weeks gestation, 80 percent of women will go into labor within twenty-four hours.

WHEN TO CALL YOUR DOCTOR

Contact your doctor if your baby stops moving or has a change in activity patterns.

If you have any vaginal bleeding, call your doctor immediately. This can be an emergency, but your doctor needs to make that decision.

Also contact your doctor if you notice leaking or gushing of fluid from the vagina.

QUESTIONS

1. *Will a contraction stress test cause me to go into labor?*
   Generally, no. The contractions are not continued for a long period of time. You will stop having contractions within an hour after the pitocin is stopped.

🌸 CHAPTER THIRTEEN

I'M RUNNING OUT OF ROOM

Ninth Lunar Month of
Pregnancy

PHYSICAL CHANGES

You'll notice an increase in the amount and thickness of your vaginal discharge. Your feet and legs will swell more at the end of the day. As you near the end of this month, you may need to limit strenuous exercise to fifteen minutes a day because you will become short of breath with less exertion. You should have gained about twenty to twenty-five pounds. The baby is bigger and has elevated your diaphragm.

By the end of this month, insomnia may have become a real problem. It may be difficult to find a comfortable sleeping position, and the baby is very active.

EMOTIONAL CHANGES

Mom

This is an exciting, happy, anxious and sad time for you. You are excited because the end seems near. At the same time, you're worried about how you will handle labor and delivery. Will the baby be all right? You wonder if you will ever get your figure back, be sexy again. You may be frightened of assuming the role of Mom, continuing your career and maintaining your role as a partner in a relationship. Can you handle everything? Of course you can! These are the normal thoughts and fears of every pregnant woman. Talk to your partner about your fears.

Dad

You probably don't understand your partner's changing moods. One minute she seems happy, the next she can't deal with things. In turn, you feel as though she couldn't understand your feelings. You wonder if you're ready to be a parent. You worry about what kind of father you will be. And always in the back of your mind is the question of how you will handle labor and delivery.

YOUR PRENATAL VISITS

You should be seen every two weeks.

What Should Be Done

Weight

Blood pressure

Urinalysis for protein and glucose

Monitoring of fetal heartbeat

Measurement of the height of the fundus

Evaluation of the size and shape of the uterus

Determination of the position of the baby

Determination of the weight of the baby

Examination of hands and feet for signs of swelling and varicose veins

Discussion of any problems or questions you both may have

Tests That May Be Done

BLOOD TEST FOR HEMOGLOBIN AND HEMATOCRIT
Pregnant women need increased amounts of iron. At this stage of pregnancy, you may need more than your vitamins and diet can give you. Your doctor will look at your hemoglobin level and determine if you need more iron.

BLOOD TEST FOR SYPHILIS
Most states require a late pregnancy test. This is usually done at thirty-six weeks.

WHAT YOU SHOULD BE DOING

This will be one of your busiest months during the pregnancy. You will need as much sleep as you can get, although it's difficult to find a comfortable position. You may want to use a "pregnant wedge," a triangular block of foam that you can lean against. Maternity shops and some home furnishing stores stock them.

You need to pack the suitcase you will be taking to the hospital. (A list of items to take is given in the appendices.) Don't forget your music box!

How will you feed your baby? Will you breast or bottle feed? You need to be comfortable with your decision. Table 13–1 may help you.

TABLE 13–1   *Breastfeeding vs. Bottle Feeding*

Breastfeeding	*Bottle Feeding*
Breast milk is perfect nutrition.	The baby may not get enough breast milk.
Breastfed babies are healthier.	The mother may have fewer breast infections.

TABLE 13–1   *Breastfeeding vs. Bottle Feeding (continued)*

The iron in breast milk is completely absorbed by the baby.	Anyone can feed the baby.
Breast milk will not cause constipation.	Some medications are passed in breast milk
Breast milk passes immunities to the baby.	The baby may go longer between feedings, thus giving the mother more time to rest.
Breastfeeding helps to develop the palate and facial muscles. There may be less tooth deacy in later life.	
Breastfeeding is more convenient, always available.	
Breastfeeding encourages maternal closeness.	
The father can give the baby a bottle of expressed breast milk.	
The mother may return to her prepregnancy weight more quickly, since breastfeeding burns calories.	

It's never too early to begin babyproofing your home. You'll find helpful guidelines in the appendices.

You and your partner need to make final arrangements for maternity/paternity leave.

You know what you would ideally like to have for your labor and delivery, but you need to make your birth plan so that everyone else knows. Use the sample birth plan on page 144 to decide on what you want.

TABLE 13–2   *Sample Birth Plan*

YES	NO	
—	—	I want to remain mobile during labor.
—	—	I want to be shaved.
—	—	I want routine IVs.
—	—	I want an enema.
—	—	I want to urinate on my own rather than be catherized.
—	—	I want spontaneous rupture of membranes.
—	—	I want an episiotomy only if necessary.
—	—	I want my partner always present.
—	—	My partner wants to cut the cord.
—	—	My partner wants to bathe the baby as soon as it is born.
—	—	I want to eat and drink during labor.
—	—	I will accept pain relief/epidural.
—	—	I want only intermittent fetal monitoring.
—	—	I want to breastfeed immediately after birth.
—	—	I do want forceps/vacuum used.
—	—	I want to use various positions for labor and delivery.

If a c-section is necessary:

—	—	I want my partner in the delivery room.
—	—	I want an epidural for anesthesia, if possible.
—	—	I want to breastfeed in the recovery room.
—	—	I want my partner to hold the baby in the delivery room.

Remember, this is an ideal birth plan. The baby, however, has not read this or discussed what he or she will do in labor.

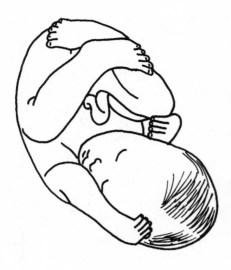

THIRTY-SIX-WEEK-OLD FETUS

You'll need help when you come home from the hospital. In earlier times, extended families lived together. Everyone helped Mom and Dad when they brought the baby home. Today, that situation usually does not exist. I encourage couples to get help for at least the first two weeks at home. This person should take care of the home, laundry, and you and your partner. You, however, should be the ones getting to know and learning to care for your baby. You need to discover your baby's personality and to continue the bonding that will begin when the baby is born.

One of the most important things you will do for your child is choosing a caregiver. If you are going to return to work, you will need to arrange for child care, either in or out of your home. Just as you intensively interviewed the pediatrician you chose, so should you screen the person or place that will care for your child. You'll find interview questions for both in-home child care and day care centers in the appendices. You'll also find a listing of resources that may help you in your search.

YOUR BABY

Your baby has started to gain about a half a pound a week. If your baby is a boy, the testes have descended into the scrotum. The baby is about seventeen to eighteen inches long and weighs between four and one half and five pounds. The baby has stopped doing flips and turns and now kicks, stretches and punches its arms and legs.

COMPLICATIONS THAT CAN OCCUR

Pregnancy-Induced Hypertension/Preeclampsia/Eclampsia/Toxemia

Preeclampsia and eclampsia, commonly referred to as pregnancy-induced hypertension (PIH) or toxemia, are toxic conditions of pregnancy characterized by high blood pressure, kidney malfunction and edema (swelling of body tissue caused by a buildup of fluid). The cause of PIH is still unknown. It is seen in varying degrees of severity and usually occurs in women pregnant for the first time.

PIH affects both the mother and the baby. The bottom number of the blood pressure reading can be 100 or more, there is protein in the urine and swelling of the hands and feet. The disease is present several weeks before any signs or symptoms are noticed. Blood flow to the kidneys, liver and uterus are decreased. Symptoms are dependent on the severity of the disease. Symptoms include protein in the urine; hypertension; headaches; changes in vision, including blurring and seeing spots and halos around objects, even complete blindness; upper abdominal pain, usually on the right side under the ribs; decrease in urination; swelling of hands and feet; and convulsions. Bleeding problems caused by a decrease in the platelet count can also be seen.

Because the flow of blood to the uterus is affected, your baby can stop growing. This condition is called intrauterine growth retardation (IUGR).

The treatment of pregnancy-induced hypertension is delivery. Your doctor will decide how to manage PIH based on the severity of the disease and the age and condition of your baby.

If your baby is thirty-seven weeks or older, your doctor will give you an IV medication to prevent or control convulsions. You may also receive a medication to control blood pressure. When blood pressure and convulsions are controlled, you will be delivered, usually vaginally.

If your baby is premature and has IUGR or is in danger and the PIH is severe, your doctor will give you medication to control convulsions and blood pressure and deliver your baby.

If your baby is premature and healthy and the PIH is mild or getting better, you will be put on bedrest and monitored closely. If you and your baby remain healthy, you will be delivered at term, usually at thirty-eight weeks. Hypertension and other symptoms are resolved after delivery.

WE'VE COME A LONG WAY

During my own pregnancy, I was admitted to the hospital well before I was due. I had been followed closely by my doctor for several weeks. During that time my blood pressure remained at 120/80; however, I gained forty pounds and my hands and face were severely swollen. I had completely stopped urinating and for several days before being admitted had noticed changes in my eyesight, including seeing silver spots. On the day I was admitted, I could barely see. My blood pressure reading was 250/140, and my doctor could not find the baby's heartbeat.

The baby had stopped moving. My doctor told me that the baby would probably not live. I was admitted to a single-bed labor room, where I underwent a three-day induction of labor with pitocin. Immediately prior to delivery, I lapsed into a coma. Several doctors, many nurses and the nun who headed the hospital were in the delivery room.

Upon awakening the next day, I was told that I had had a beautiful, but tiny, baby girl. I couldn't believe it, because I had been told my baby would not live. But when the nurse brought in a tiny, red-faced bundle, I knew that this was my baby.

I was discharged with my premature miracle baby five days later and was on bedrest for several weeks after delivery. My daughter grew into the beautiful mother of my grandson.

This type of management simply doesn't happen today. My doctor gave me excellent care almost thirty years ago, but we've come a long way.

Intrauterine Growth Retardation (IUGR)

Babies who grow slowly or who stop growing in utero and when born are at or below the tenth percentile have intrauterine growth retardation (IUGR). There are two types of IUGR: asymmetric IUGR, in which the body slows or stops growth but the head continues to grow; and symmetric IUGR, in which the entire baby stops or slows growth.

Asymmetric IUGR can be caused by pregnancy-induced hypertension, kidney disease and heavy smoking. It usually occurs at approximately twenty-six to thirty-six weeks.

Symmetric IUGR begins much earlier and can be caused by genetic abnormalities; developmental abnormalities; infections such as rubella, toxoplasmosis, herpes and CMV; maternal heart disease; and heavy smoking throughout pregnancy.

The first sign of IUGR is slow increase or no increase in fundal height. If this occurs, your doctor will order a sonogram to make the diagnosis. The amount of amniotic fluid will also be assessed. You will then have a non-stress test and a biophysical profile to evaluate the baby. If there is a good amount of fluid and the baby is healthy, you may be monitored closely and put on bedrest. You will have an NST and BPP twice a week. If the baby grows, you will be monitored closely and delivered when the baby's lungs are mature.

If there is a decreased amount of fluid and the baby is not healthy, you may be delivered immediately.

Oligohydramnios

Oligohydramnios is a decrease in the amount of amniotic fluid around the baby. The normal amount of fluid is about a liter. The first indication of this condition may be a decrease in the fundal height, or no increase in fundal height. The diagnosis is made on sonogram. Abnormal urinary tract (kidneys, ureters, bladder and urethra) development, slow leaking of amniotic fluid, intrauterine growth retardation and postdate pregnancy all can be causes of this condition. Depending on the cause of the oligohydramnios, your doctor will either monitor you and your baby closely or deliver the baby.

Polyhydramnios

Polyhydramnios is an abnormal increase in the amount of amniotic fluid. The first indication that this condition is present is an abnormal increase in the fundal height. Your doctor will make the diagnosis based on measurements obtained on sonogram. These measurements, called the amniotic fluid index, will assess the severity of the increase in fluid volume. Polyhydramnios is associated with maternal diabetes; erythroblastosis fetalis, a condition that occurs in babies whose mothers have Rh iso-immunization; multiple gestation; and abnormal organ system development, including the brain and spinal cord, the gastrointestinal tract and the heart. No reason for this condition is found in 35 percent of cases.

Your doctor will try to find the cause. You and your baby will be monitored closely and delivered either when the baby's lungs are mature or if the baby becomes unhealthy.

Polyhydramnios can cause premature labor, ineffective labor contractions and postpartum hemorrhage.

WHEN TO CALL YOUR DOCTOR

Contact your doctor if you have a headache that doesn't go away with acetaminophen, relaxation or meditation; if you notice a pain on the right side of your abdomen under your ribs; if you notice a decrease in urination in either volume or frequency; if you notice swelling of your hands and face; or if you begin to have changes in vision, such as blurring or seeing spots or halos.

QUESTIONS

1. Do all headaches mean that I may have PIH?

No, only headaches associated with hypertension and swelling of your hands and feet may be associated with PIH.

CHAPTER FOURTEEN

ISN'T IT TIME YET?

Tenth Lunar Month

PHYSICAL CHANGES

You will notice that breathing is easier, because the baby has dropped or engaged. This means the head or buttocks are now in the pelvis. However, as your breathing becomes easier, the pelvic pressure has increased. You now are urinating more frequently due to the pressure of the baby on your bladder. The baby is kicking and punching more, but the large movements have decreased. You may notice more Braxton-Hicks contractions during this last month. There is an increase in fatigue because you are not sleeping well. It is difficult to find a comfortable position. Leg cramps may have increased. Your appetite may be either increased or decreased. Each woman is different and each pregnancy is different with respect to appetite.

EMOTIONAL CHANGES

Mom

Your dreams have increased in number. They can be wonderful visions of how pretty and beautiful your baby is, or they can be nightmares that something happens to the baby. There are many theories for why mothers have dreams of losing their babies. However, none seem to answer the question. What is known is that dreams mean nothing in predicting the outcome for your baby.

You have some sense of relief that the pregnancy is almost over, but you're still concerned about how you will do in labor and de-

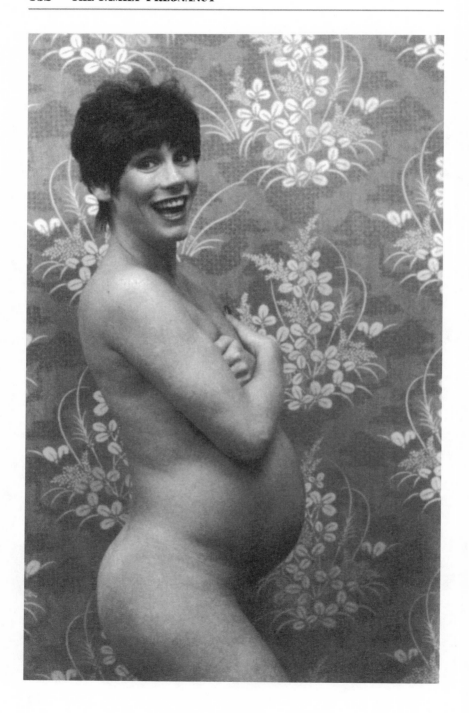

livery. You may become more restless and irritable before delivery. Isn't it time yet, you wonder. Some women during this month "feather the nest." You may have a burst of energy and clean everything in sight. I've had patients who did the laundry, cleaned the house, rewashed and folded the baby's clothes, then came into the office and announced it was time to have the baby.

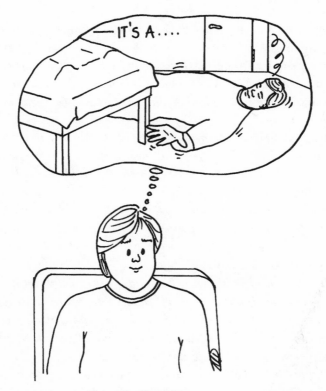

Every Dad's nightmare . . .

Dad

You may be feeling an increased anxiety about the labor and delivery. Will you faint? Will you be a good coach? You may worry about whether your partner and baby will be all right. You may even feel left out of the whole thing, since everyone is paying attention to mom. You may also be worried about getting to the hospital on time. These are normal emotions and are shared by most fathers.

You may even be worried about whether you will care for the baby. What if you don't like it? Stay calm.

I'M NOT GOING TO STAY

Jonathan had been quick to tell me at the first prenatal visit that he was not going to be in the room when the baby was delivered. Although he attended prepared childbirth classes with his wife, Diana, he continued to inform me that he was not staying for labor or birth. I never contradicted him or told him he had to stay. He just wanted me to know that he wasn't doing it.

Diana went into labor in the middle of the night. I met them at the hospital, examined Diana and told them it would be a few hours before baby Zoe made her debut. Jonathan said he would stay a little while, "until Diana has more pain, then I'm leaving. I don't want to see her in pain." Diana did well through the first stage of labor, and Jonathan was a great coach. When Diana was ready to deliver, I informed Jonathan. "I'll stay, but I don't want to see anything," he said. "I don't want to know if the baby is all right."

After Zoe made her way into the world, I asked Jonathan if he would like to introduce his daughter to her mother. I looked up to see tears running down his face, as he watched his baby daughter in wonder. I wrapped the baby and handed her to him. Diana was settled and I had to leave the room to attend to another patient.

I returned a few hours later to find father and daughter deep in conversation. Diana was pleading, "Please let me hold her a little while. I'll give her back." Diana then looked at me and said that her husband had not relinquished the baby since birth.

YOUR PRENATAL VISITS

You should be seen weekly.

What Should Be Done

Weight

Blood pressure

Urinalysis for protein and glucose

Monitoring of fetal heartbeat

Measurement of the height of the fundus

Evaluation of the size and shape of the uterus

Determination of the position of the baby

Determination of the weight of the baby

Evaluation to check for engagement of the baby's head into the pelvis

Examination of hands and feet for varicose veins

Cervical examination beginning at thirty-eight to forty weeks

Discussion of any problems or questions you both may have

Discussion of your birth plan

Discussion of the signs of labor

Discussion of when to call the doctor

WHAT YOU SHOULD BE DOING

If you're still working, you should be making final plans to take leave when the baby is born. Some women work until delivery. If you feel well, there's no reason that you can't; however, long-distance travel should be curtailed.

You should purchase a safety car seat this month. Car seats are required by law and you cannot take the baby home from the hospital without one. (See the appendices for more information.)

Try to stay comfortable and calm. Everyone will ask you when you're having the baby. Just tell them the baby hasn't confided that information to you.

Make final arrangements for any help you'll need when you come home. Make sure the baby nurse, if you're using one, is notified. Make a list of people who need to be called, and pack it in your suitcase.

If you have older children, discuss your upcoming trip to the hospital. If they've attended sibling classes, they'll be better prepared. Reassure them that they will be able to visit you and the new baby in the hospital. You may want to arrange for them to stay overnight with friends or family when you have the baby.

RELAX.

YOUR BABY

Your baby now weighs between six and one half and eight and one half pounds. Its head or bottom is engaged in the pelvis. The baby may have a little or a great deal of hair. Its fingernails need a manicure. The baby is kicking and poking. There is no room to do somersaults anymore, but it is still active.

COMPLICATIONS THAT CAN OCCUR

Postdate Pregnancy

A postdate pregnancy is one that goes beyond forty-two weeks. Up to 12 percent of pregnancies can go beyond the forty-second week. There is an increase in intrauterine death, as much as four to six times the normal number, for pregnancies that go to forty-three or forty-four weeks.

Complications for the mother in postdate pregnancy include an increased c-section rate because of the size of the baby; postpartum hemorrhage due to uterine atony, in which the uterus does not contract and remains flaccid after delivery of a large baby; and increased number of vaginal and rectal tears.

Complications for the baby include damage to the placenta, which does not supply enough oxygen and nutrients to the baby; increased incidence of birth trauma, such as shoulder dystocia, in which the shoulders of the baby become stuck in the birth channel; increased risk of intrauterine death; suffocation from meconium, the first bowel movement a baby makes (babies who are stressed will move their bowels while in the uterus); and postmaturity syndrome. Postmaturity syndrome includes muscle wasting; long fingernails; peeling skin; meconium staining; decreased amniotic fluid; and macrosomia, or abnormally large size for the gestational age. Babies can also develop a condition called meconium aspiration if they breathe the meconium into their lungs.

At forty-one weeks, your doctor will begin fetal testing with NSTs and biophysical profiles. He or she will probably induce labor by forty-two weeks. If your cervix is not ready, a gel will be used to help soften it. If your cervix does not soften, your doctor may choose to perform a c-section, especially if there is decreased amniotic fluid and a nonreactive NST.

Abruptio Placentae

0.5 to 1.5 percent of all pregnancies have a separation of the placenta from the uterus before the baby is born. This is called abruptio placentae. The symptoms can range from mild bleeding with or without pain to severe pain and hemorrhaging. Mild abruptio may involve only a small portion of the placenta. If you are premature, you will be observed in the hospital until time of delivery. If you are ready to deliver, you will probably be delivered vaginally. If there is a significant portion of the placenta separated, placing your baby in jeopardy, you will have an emergency c-section and blood replacement as necessary.

WHEN TO CALL YOUR DOCTOR

Contact your doctor if you notice abdominal pain and bleeding, if your membranes rupture (water breaks) or if you are in labor.

QUESTIONS

1. *What starts labor?*

We don't know exactly what starts labor, but we do know that it is an intricate interaction of the fetus, amniotic fluid and membranes. A newly discovered compound found in the amniotic fluid is believed to come from fetal urine. This compound combines with calcium to activate a chemical that is released from the membranes. This chemical is activated to prostaglandin. Prostaglandin plays an important role in initiating labor. There is also an increase in the number of oxytocin receptors in the uterus. Oxytocin is a substance that is released by the brain to start contractions. This substance finds its way to the uterus through the bloodstream. The receptors are waiting and contractions begin. A special substance that keeps the uterus relaxed appears to decrease as labor starts.

2. *What is engagement?*

Engagement is when the baby's head or bottom goes into the pelvis and is in the birth position.

3. *If I have herpes, will I have to have a c-section?*

Not necessarily. If you do not have active lesions, you can have a vaginal delivery. However, if you do have active lesions, you will require a c-section. Herpes can cause blindness if a baby passes through a vagina with active lesions.

4. What is a VBAC? If I have had a previous c-section, do I need another one?

Vaginal birth after cesarean, or VBAC, is a routine procedure today. At one time if you had one c-section, every baby after that was born by c-section. Vaginal delivery after a low-transverse c-section is safe. A transverse incision is made low on the uterus in a horizontal manner. Even if you have had two c-sections you may be a candidate for VBAC. The risk of uterine rupture of the previous scar is 0.5 percent. About 30 percent of all c-sections done in this country are repeat c-sections. If everyone who had one had tried for a VBAC, we could greatly decrease the number of c-sections done in the United States. From 50 to 85 percent of women who try for VBAC are successful in delivering vaginally. The only contraindication to a VBAC is a previous c-section with a classical incision. This means that the uterine incision was made vertically, high on the uterus. The risk of rupture after a classical c-section is 4 percent or greater. To be a candidate for VBAC, you must have one fetus, a previous low-transverse uterine incision and a normal current pregnancy. A physician capable of doing operative deliveries should be available.

VBAC is now considered routine and treated the same as any other vaginal delivery.

5. How do I know if I'm in labor?

There is a difference between false labor and real labor. the table below can help you distinguish between the two:

TABLE 14-1 *Is It Labor?*

	Real Labor	False Labor
Bloody show	YES	NO

TABLE 14–1 *(cont.)*	*Real Labor*	*False Labor*
Loss of mucus plug*	YES	NO
Cervix effaces	YES	NO
Cervix dilates	YES	NO
Membranes rupture	YES	NO
Contractions are regular	YES	NO
Contractions increase in strength	YES	NO
Contractions increase in duration	YES	NO
Contractions increase in frequency	YES	NO
Contractions go away with activity	YES	NO
Contractions go away with a warm bath	NO	YES
Contractions go away with a glass of wine	NO	YES

This chart may help you distinguish real labor from false labor.

*May be expelled before labor begins

6. When do I call the doctor?

Your doctor may have different protocols about when he or she wants to hear from you. Definitely call if your membranes rupture. You should have regular contractions. Your doctor will want to know the frequency and duration of the contractions, and how long they have been regular.

7. If I need pain relief, what is available to me? What anesthesia is available?

The most commonly used drugs for pain relief in labor are Demerol and Nubain. Both can be given through an IV or by injection in the buttocks. Demerol causes a little more respiratory depression in the baby. This means that the baby may not want to breathe. The baby may also be sleepy and

CONTRACTIONS

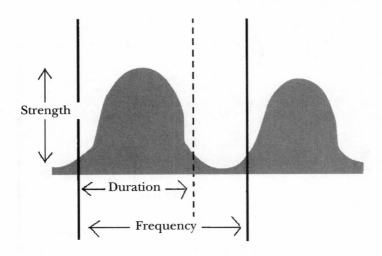

DURATION is measured from the beginning to the end of one contraction.

FREQUENCY is measured from the beginning of one contraction to the beginning of the next.

STRENGTH indicates how strong the contraction is.

won't be able to suck well. Remember, whatever you take goes to your baby. The baby is not able to clear drugs as quickly as you do. Any drug can make you dizzy or drowsy, and cause nausea and vomiting.

Obstetric anesthesia is available. The various types of anesthesia are paracervical block, pudendal block, local perineal anesthesia, spinal block and epidural.

EPIDURAL ANESTHESIA

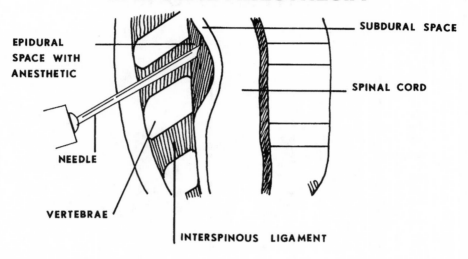

EPIDURAL
SPACE WITH
ANESTHETIC

SUBDURAL SPACE

SPINAL CORD

NEEDLE

VERTEBRAE

INTERSPINOUS LIGAMENT

A paracervical block is used for delivery when forceps or a vacuum must be used. Local anesthesia is injected around the cervix to numb the nerves that go to the perineum. A paracervical block can cause the baby's heart rate to decrease.

A pudendal block also uses local anesthesia techniques. It is injected in a similar fashion as the paracervical and also numbs the pain fibers to the perineum. It is used for forceps and vacuum deliveries and when an episiotomy must be made.

Local perineal anesthesia is anesthesia injected directly into the perineum. This is used before an episiotomy is made.

Spinal anesthesia is local anesthesia injected into the spine. An IV will be placed in your arm and you will be given about a liter of fluid. Then you will sit up, hunched over a table. Your back will be washed with surgical soap. A fine needle will be inserted between the bones of your spine into the fluid that surrounds the spinal cord and a small amount of spinal fluid removed. An equal amount of anesthetic will

be added. You will then be placed on your back with a pillow under your left hip to displace the uterus from your
back. Spinal anesthesia works immediately, but it lasts only
about an hour. The complications of spinal anesthesia include a drop in blood pressure and a "spinal headache,"
which can last up to a week.

Epidural anesthesia is the method of choice for many doctors for labor and delivery. It is safe for the baby. The complications for the mother include a drop in blood pressure,
allergic reactions to the medication, "spinal headache," a
true spinal block and occasionally slowed labor. Epidural
anesthesia does not increase your chances of having a c-section or forceps delivery.

An IV will be started and you will be given a liter of fluid.
You will then be asked to curl up into a ball, or to sit up,
hunched over a table. Your back will be washed with surgical soap. A needle will then be inserted between the vertebrae into the epidural space and a small amount of medication will be injected. This is a test dose to make sure that the
needle has not entered a blood vessel or the spinal fluid. If
the placement is proper, a tiny catheter is threaded through
the needle, and the needle is removed. The catheter is
taped in place. You will then be positioned on your back,
with a pillow under your left hip. The catheter will be attached to a pump that will deliver a small, continuous dose
of medication. This is called a continuous epidural and involves a dilute solution of the medication. The catheter can
also be attached to a syringe that contains the medication.
You will receive bolus doses when you begin to feel pain.

An epidural relaxes the pelvic muscles and the nerves are
bathed in the local anesthetic medication. You will still feel
the pressure of the contractions and the urge to push. The
catheter is removed after the baby is born.

CHAPTER FIFTEEN

PLEASE STOP FOR THE RED LIGHTS ON THE WAY TO THE HOSPITAL

Labor and Delivery

⚛ LABOR CAN BE DEFINED AS REPETITIVE UTERINE contractions that open the cervix and allow delivery of the baby, placenta and membranes. Labor is divided into three stages: dilation and effacement of the cervix, delivery of the baby and delivery of the placenta.

POSITION OF THE BABY

Babies present in different positions. This means that the presenting part is the part of the baby that is over the cervix.

VERTEX

About 95 percent of babies present with their face toward the mother's spine. The majority of these have their chin tucked into the chest. This position of the head is called occiput anterior, meaning that the occipital bone, a bone at the back of the skull, is facing forward. The rest of vertex babies are born "sunny side up," or looking up at the ceiling. They face forward in the uterus. Heads in this position are called occiput posterior.

BREECH

Some 3 to 4 percent of babies are born buttocks first. The legs of these babies can be in several positions.

Frank

Both legs are straight up in front of the body, with the feet alongside the baby's head in the frank breech position. The baby in this position can be delivered vaginally as long as additional conditions are met.

Complete

The breech baby in this position is sitting Indian-style with the ankles crossed.

Incomplete (Footling)

The baby is sitting in the same position as above but with one foot extended into the vagina.

Criteria for Delivery

Certain conditions must be met to safely deliver a breech baby (see Table 15–1). Although problems can be encountered, a frank breech delivery is safe in experienced hands.

TABLE 15–1   *Conditions for a Vaginal Breech Delivery*

Your baby must be in the frank breech position.

You must be at least thirty-six weeks pregnant.

Your baby must weigh between five and one half and seven and one half pounds.

You must have had a normal, uncomplicated pregnancy.

You must not have any medical problems.

The baby's head must be in the right position.

The buttocks must be engaged.

You must have adequate pelvic bone measurements.

Your doctor has informed you of the risks.

Version

If your baby is breech, your doctor could suggest turning him into a head-down position. To do this, you must be at thirty-seven to thirty-nine weeks. You also should have no medical problems or any complications of pregnancy; your membranes should be intact and you should not be in labor; there should be only one baby and the presenting part should not be engaged; and you should have no history of previous uterine surgery or bleeding at the end of pregnancy.

You will be admitted to the labor floor and given an IV solution containing a tocolytic, the same medication used to stop premature labor. The baby's heart rate will be monitored. Your doctor will place his or her hands on the baby's buttocks and head. Using a forward or backward motion, your doctor will slowly attempt to turn the baby 180 degrees. An ultrasound will be done to confirm the success of the version.

Approximately 70 percent of version attempts are successful.

Other

Besides vertex and breech, babies also present with other fetal parts first. These can be face, brow, shoulder or any other part of the body. Some babies have a hand on top of their head. This is called a compound presentation.

If the baby is lying across the uterus, in a transverse presentation, your doctor may attempt a version.

FIRST STAGE OF LABOR

The first stage involves dilation, which is the opening of the cervix, and effacement, which is the thinning of the cervix. Membranes may rupture at any time before, during or after this stage.

FIRST STAGE OF LABOR

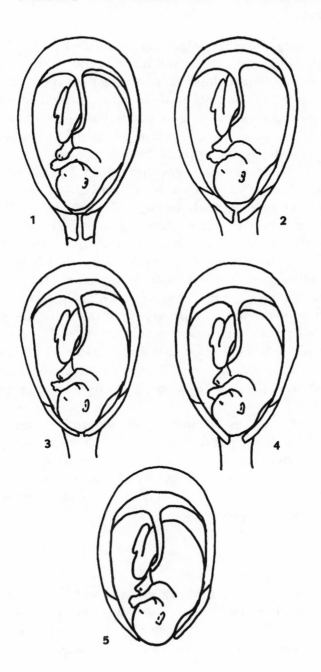

Latent Phase

The beginning of the first stage of labor is called the latent phase. During this time, your cervix will dilate to four centimeters and efface. You may have a bloody show during this phase. This is mucus and a small amount of blood mixed together. You may have lost your mucus plug, the plug of mucus that keeps the cervix impenetrable, up to two weeks before the latent phase begins. It may also pass during latent phase labor.

Latent phase labor may begin with a backache, diarrhea, frequent soft bowel movements or menstruallike cramps. The cramps will begin irregularly, lasting a short duration. They may begin about twenty to thirty minutes apart, but they may be so mild that you won't notice them. As the contractions become closer and more intense, you should begin timing them. You should not be alone and may want to be active. Moving around and doing things will help the time pass quickly. You should eat lightly, but do eat. Also, be sure to keep yourself hydrated. Drink as much as you are comfortable taking.

Latent phase is the longest of the two phases of the first stage of labor. It usually lasts eight to eighteen hours for a first-time pregnancy (nullipara), six to twelve hours for a repeat pregnancy (multipara).

As the contractions become closer and more intense, your cervix will be dilating and effacing. When contractions are approximately five minutes apart and last sixty seconds, you are close to or in active-phase labor. You should call your doctor, if you have not already done so. Remember to take your suitcase with you to the birthing site.

Active Phase

When you arrive at the birthing site, you will be assessed as to whether you are in actual labor. The baby will be monitored for a period of time. You will have a pelvic exam to check the dilation and effacement of the cervix. Your blood pressure should be taken. Your partner may be asked to wait in another area while you're being evaluated.

If you're in labor, you will be taken to a birthing or labor room. Make sure your partner is notified if he has been asked to wait. During the active phase, your contractions will become closer and more intense. Your cervix will dilate to ten centimeters and be completely effaced. You will use all the techniques you've learned in your prepared childbirth classes to cope with labor.

The most intense period in active labor is called transition. This is when your cervix dilates from seven to nine centimeters. Transition can last from one and one half to two and one half hours. You may have difficulty concentrating on your labor techniques. Your partner should be coaching and encouraging you.

The active phase is much shorter than the latent phase, lasting from two to six hours in nullipara, from less than an hour to four hours in multipara.

Your doctor may perform an amniotomy, or artificial rupture of the membranes, if your membranes have not ruptured on their own. This, however, may not be done until the end of the first stage of labor.

If you can tolerate movement and the baby is healthy, you should move as much as possible while you're in labor. Gravity and movement help nature. If your baby is healthy and no problems have developed, it may be monitored only intermittently.

Different positions may help with the pain. Table 15–2 lists some of the positions you could try.

TABLE 15–2   *Positions for Labor*

FIRST STAGE

STANDING   Helps work with gravity; contractions less
                  painful; helps backache; may speed labor;
                  aligns the baby with the pelvic angle; could
                  become tiring, but less tiring if you lean
                  forward supported by partner.

TABLE 15–2 (*cont.*)

WALKING	Same advantages as standing, plus may encourage descent of the presenting part.
SITTING	Works with gravity; may be able to rest; sitting cross-legged may open pelvic outlet; fetal monitoring possible; can slow labor after a long period.
HANDS AND KNEES	Helps relieve back pain; may rotate posterior baby; tiring for long periods.
KNEES, CHEST SUPPORTED	Same as hands and knees, but less strain on arms.
SEMI-SITTING	Same as sitting; increases back pain.
LYING ON SIDE	Lowers blood pressure; excellent resting position; contractions may be longer.
LYING ON BACK	Least effective for progress of labor; may become hypotensive and the baby may become distressed; may increase backache; fetal monitoring can be done.

SECOND STAGE

FORTY-FIVE-DEGREE ANGLE (Legs pulled back and shoulders elevated)	Widens pelvic outlet; uses gravity to some extent; better for backache than lying down; may work well with epidural.

TABLE 15–2 (*cont.*)

LYING ON SIDE	Lowers blood pressure; eases backache; easier to relax between pushes.
HANDS AND KNEES	Excellent for rotating posterior baby; reduces backache.
SQUATTING	Uses gravity to help the baby descend and rotate; partner can support your back and arms; widens pelvic outlet.
LITHOTOMY	Lying back with legs in stirrups; good for forceps or vacuum, extensive episiotomy, delivery of breech.
SEMILITHOTOMY	Same as lithotomy, with head and shoulders elevated.

LABOR AND DELIVERY IN WATER

Labor in water may ease contractions and gentle delivery. It is not available at all facilities. It has been found to be safe for the baby, and may lower blood pressure in the mother. The usual position is semi-sitting with your partner behind you, supporting you.

Pain Control

This is what you have been working toward—labor and delivery. You have chosen your method of labor and childbirth and have practiced, and now you must put it all to use. Remember your breathing and focusing techniques. If you're experiencing a severe backache during labor, your baby may be posterior. To help relieve the pain, your partner can roll a tennis ball in the small of your back. Massage and meditation are wonderful ways to relax between contractions.

If you're unable to maintain concentration or if the pain has become more intense than you can tolerate, medications and anesthesia are available. This doesn't mean that you're a failure, just that labor may be difficult or more intense than usual. Everyone has her own level of pain tolerance.

THE IDEAL LABOR

Linda and Robert had an uneventful, normal pregnancy. Linda had developed no complications and had gained twenty-eight pounds. Robert had gained only ten pounds. Linda began latent phase labor at three in the afternoon, while at work. It began as a mild backache and cramping. Linda went home and checked her hospital bag. She packed the baby's music box. She then began to clean the apartment. Robert came in as Linda was having a mild contraction. She looked up at him and said it was almost time to call the doctor. Linda continued to drink fluids as the evening progressed, and at eleven o'clock she decided it was time to go to the hospital. Her contractions were five minutes apart and were lasting sixty seconds. The couple called me and told me the timing of Linda's contractions. I said I would meet them at the hospital.

COMPLICATIONS OF FIRST STAGE

Prolonged Latent Phase

A latent phase that lasts longer than twenty hours in nullipara and fourteen hours in multipara may be prolonged. You should call your doctor if contractions don't become closer. Your doctor may prescribe a sedative, which may have one of three effects: When you awaken, you may be in active labor, you may have stopped contracting, or you may still be having the same contractions. If you are in active labor, your labor will progress. If you stop contracting, you were in false labor. If your contractions are the same, your doctor may decide to admit you to the hospital and augment your labor, or add to your spontaneous contractions, with pitocin.

Prolonged Active Phase

When cervical dilation stops or slows, it is called a prolonged active phase. If this occurs, your doctor may augment your labor with pitocin.

Precipitate Labor

This is labor that lasts three hours or less, from first contraction to delivery of the baby. While this sounds wonderful, it does present problems. The contractions may be fast and intense immediately. You could be overwhelmed by this. You should go to your birthing site as soon as possible. Sometimes the baby does not wait until you leave home or until you arrive at the birthing site. You will then be faced with an emergency delivery. This is every new father's worst nightmare. Don't panic; just follow the directions for an emergency delivery (see Table 15–3).

TABLE 15–3   *Emergency Delivery*

WHEN BABY WON'T WAIT

If you're at home or on the way to the hospital, contractions may begin coming very hard and very fast. You may soon feel the overwhelming urge to push. Try panting breaths. This may work for a short period of time, which may be long enough for help to arrive. If you're alone, call for help. DO NOT TRY TO DRIVE A CAR YOURSELF. If you're at home, you or your partner should call for medical aid. If you're in the car, have your partner pull over to the side of the road.

Mom

Take off your clothes below the waist, if you have time. Lie in a comfortable position. Do not push. This may cause you to tear. You will feel a burning sensation as the baby's head stretches your vagina.

Dad

KEEP CALM. Have cloth towels, clothing, paper towels or tissues ready. Wash your hands, if possible.

TABLE 15–3 (*cont.*)

DELIVERY OF THE BABY: You will see the top of the baby's head as it stretches the vagina. As the baby's head delivers, support it. Gently wipe the baby's face. If the membranes are intact, open them with your fingernail and push them away from the baby's face. Feel around the baby's neck for the umbilical cord. If one is present, slip it over the baby's head. Have your partner gently push to deliver the baby's body. Hold the baby securely; remember, the baby will be wet and slippery. Quickly wipe the baby clean and hand him to his mother. Most babies cry within a few seconds of birth. If the baby does not cry, place him across her abdomen, head down, and gently rub his back. This will usually start his breathing. After the baby begins to breathe, hand him to his mother.

DELIVERY OF THE PLACENTA: DO NOT CUT THE CORD. DO NOT PULL ON THE CORD. The placenta will deliver on its own, usually a few minutes after the baby. After the placenta delivers, wrap it up. Bleeding is normal. Your partner will lose a few cups of blood. Bleeding will slow greatly after the placenta is delivered. Cover mother and baby.

AFTER THE DELIVERY

Mom

Place the baby on your chest, skin to skin. This will keep the baby warm. After the placenta has delivered, place the baby to the breast to suck. This will release oxytocin and contract the uterus. If the baby will not suck, gently massage your nipples. Massage the uterus in a circular motion until you feel it become firm.

Keep the baby warm and covered, especially the baby's head. The baby loses heat from his head. Talk to your baby.

Dad

If you're at home, get to know your baby and wait for the ambulance to arrive. If you're in the car, drive to the hospital.

Prolapsed Cord

If your membranes rupture and the presenting part of the baby is not engaged, the cord could come out. This is an emergency. A prolapsed cord will shut off the oxygen supply to the baby. If you are at home and you feel the pulsing cord between your legs, get into a knee-chest position with your buttocks elevated and have your partner call for help. If you're on the way to the hospital, get into the back seat as quickly as possible and assume a knee-chest position. When you reach the hospital, have your partner go for help. If this happens at the hospital, you will be told to get into the knee-chest position. You will be delivered by emergency cesarean section.

Arrest of Labor

This is when dilation and effacement stop despite contractions that are frequent enough and strong enough. Your doctor will do a cesarean delivery.

Chorioamnionitis

Chorioamnionitis is an infection of the fluid or membranes. You will develop a fever and uterine tenderness in labor. The baby's heart rate will increase. If you are close to delivery, your doctor may elect to wait to give you antibiotics. This is so that cultures on the baby will not be falsely negative. If you are not close to delivery, your doctor may start IV antibiotics.

INDUCTION OF LABOR

Induction of labor is contractions started by artificial means rather than spontaneously for the purpose of delivery. Table 15–4 lists reasons that labor may be induced.

TABLE 15–4   *Induction of Labor*

INDICATIONS

Preeclampsia	Diabetes
Eclampsia	Postdate pregnancy
Premature rupture of membranes	Chronic hypertension
	Kidney disease
Chorioamnionitis	Rh iso-immunization
Abruptio placentae (partial)	Impending fetal distress
Fetal death	

CONTRAINDICATIONS

Previous classical cesarean section	Cephalo-pelvic disproportion
	Invasive cervical cancer
Previous myomectomy, if extensive	Placenta previa
Abnormal presentation of baby	Active herpes infection

When you report to the labor floor, you will be taken to a birthing or labor room. After the baby is monitored, an IV will be started containing pitocin, a medication that causes contractions. Pitocin will be increased periodically until you have contractions approximately every three minutes. These contractions will continue until delivery. The baby will be monitored throughout labor.

If you and the baby are healthy and if your membranes are accessible, your doctor may elect to rupture them. You may be allowed to walk, sit or lie in bed at your option. 75 percent of women will begin labor spontaneously within a few hours of membrane rupture. If contractions do not begin spontaneously, you will be given pitocin.

SECOND STAGE OF LABOR: DELIVERY OF THE BABY

This is when you will appreciate being in great shape. Your exercise program has built stamina. You are about to do the hardest work you have ever done: pushing your baby into the world. The position you choose should be comfortable for you (see pages 169–171). This stage lasts from thirty minutes to two hours in nullipara, five to sixty minutes in multipara. If you are doing well and the baby is healthy, you may push much longer than the usual time as long as you are making progress. You may have an absence of contractions for a brief period of time as you begin the second stage. This is normal and allows you to regain some strength.

Delivery of Vertex

As your baby's head descends into the vagina, you will feel the urge to push. Listen to your body. Relax as much as possible and push, using the same muscles you use to have a bowel movement. Do not push when you are not having contractions. You need the force of the contractions to effectively help your baby descend. Between contractions and pushing, try to let your body relax as much as possible. As your baby nears the perineum, you will feel a burning sensation. You have to push past this. As you do, the top of the baby's head will be seen. This is called crowning. Your caregiver may use mineral oil to massage and stretch your perineum. Work with your contractions to allow the baby's head to stretch the perineum.

If you are tearing, the baby is having problems or you are having problems, your doctor may perform an episiotomy. An episiotomy is a cut made in the perineum to enlarge the vaginal opening. There is a great deal of controversy over the need for this. You should discuss this with your doctor before labor.

As your baby's head is delivered, it will rotate to one side or the other. Your doctor will suction the baby's nose and mouth free of mucus. He or she will then check the baby's neck for a cord and

EPISIOTOMY

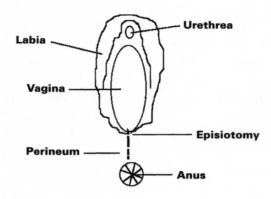

if one is present will slip it over the baby's head. The doctor will ask you to push gently, and the baby's body will be delivered. He or she will then clamp the cord in two places and may ask your partner to cut between the two clamps. Depending on the method of birth you have chosen, the baby will be given to your partner to bathe or place on your stomach.

Touch your baby and talk to her. Your partner should also touch and talk to the baby. Get to know her. Let her know who you are as you welcome her into the world.

Delivery of Breech

Because the baby's body is much softer than its head, you will not have to push as hard. You will most likely have an epidural. Your doctor will do an episiotomy and ask you to push gently to allow the buttocks to deliver. After the buttocks and hips are delivered, the doctor will reach into the vagina and deliver first one leg, then the other. He or she will wrap the baby's hips and legs in a towel and allow the body to deliver spontaneously. When the body has delivered to the shoulders, the doctor will reach into the vagina and deliver each arm. The baby's head may deliver spontaneously. If it doesn't, the doctor will place fingers over the baby's face, one on each side of the baby's nostrils. He or she will do a maneuver that will allow the head to deliver. Sometimes forceps need to be applied to deliver the head without trauma.

The cord is then clamped and cut.

Apgar Score

When your baby is one minute and five minutes old, he will be given a score that reflects how well he is doing. A usual Apgar score is 8/9 or 9/9. Points are usually taken off for the baby's color (see Table 15–5).

TABLE 15–5   *Apgar Scoring System**

Sign	0	1	2
RESPIRATORY EFFORT	None	Slow, irregular breathing; weak cry	Strong cry; regular breathing
HEART RATE	None	Less than 100 beats per minute	Good, over 100 beats per minute
COLOR	Blue, pale	Body pink, hands and feet bluish	Completely pink, including extremities
MUSCLE TONE	Limp, flaccid	Some flexing of extremities, fingers and toes	Active movement of all extremities
RESPONSE TO STIMULI (REFLEX)	No response	Grimace	Cry

*Apgar scores, an indication of your baby's well-being, are based on the above parameters. They are given at one minute and five minutes after birth.

THE PERFECT DELIVERY

Linda and Robert arrived at the hospital a few minutes before I did. Robert was pale, but otherwise in great shape. Linda was dealing with the contractions quite well. She was admitted to a birthing room. The lights were lowered and the CDs they brought were popped into the player. Linda's blood pressure was taken and information such as gravity, the number of pregnancies she had had, and parity, the number of live births she had had, was obtained by the nurse who would be with her and Robert during labor. I examined her and found her cervix to be six centimeters dilated and the baby descended to a good position. After assessing the baby on the monitor for about twenty minutes and ascertaining the baby was healthy, Linda was allowed to get out of bed. She walked and rocked for a few hours, resting on her left side when she tired. Robert reminded her to focus and visualize, taking slow, deep breaths with each contraction. When she lost her concentration and relaxation during transition, Linda stood under a warm shower, with the water hitting the small of her back. This seemed to help, and she was able to return to breathing and visualizing. During her resting periods the baby was monitored and found to be doing well. Linda had continued to drink fluids throughout her labor.

When she reached complete dilation, Linda felt the urge to push. She wanted to deliver in the squatting position. A squatting bar was placed over her head. Robert sat behind her and supported her back. She was elevated so that her feet were about twelve inches off the floor. I sat cross-legged on the floor, assessing her perineum with each push. As she began to feel a burning, I saw the baby's head crown. I asked Robert to support her and she leaned back into a semi-squatting position. The next contraction brought the baby's head. I suctioned the mouth and nose and felt for a cord. Linda then gently pushed the baby's body out. I clamped the cord and lifted the baby so that Robert could cut the cord.

Robert then helped Linda to lie back on the bed. I handed him his lovely baby girl to bathe. As I turned to attend to Linda, Robert asked me, "How long do I keep her head under water?" I whirled around to find Dad waiting for an answer. I then told him to keep the baby's head out of water and just give her a bath, which I assisted him in doing. As he lavished water over his daughter, he spoke to her gently. We dried the baby and wrapped her in warm blankets; then Robert introduced her to her mother. They looked at the baby and declared they had just decided on a name: Kathleen Mary, the middle name after me. It was the first time a baby had been named for me.

COMPLICATIONS OF SECOND STAGE

Arrest of Descent
Arrest of descent means that the baby's head does not descend or descends only part of the way. If the baby's head is low enough in the vagina, your doctor may apply forceps to assist the descent and deliver the baby. Forceps look like large curved salad spoons. Today, forceps are applied only if the head is very low or crowning. You will require anesthesia for forceps application. Your doctor may use a paracervical block or a pudendal block if you do not have an epidural. He or she will then empty your bladder. Forceps will be applied one at a time. With the next contraction after application, the doctor will pull as you push. Forceps application is becoming a lost art, so ask about your doctor's experience in forceps deliveries.

Another method of assisted delivery is vacuum extraction. A silastic cup is applied to the top of the baby's head and a low-level suction vacuum is established. The doctor will pull as you push with each contraction. The same rules apply to vacuum as to forceps.

If the head is too high in the birth canal to do an assisted delivery, a cesarean section will be done.

Shoulder Dystocia
Shoulder dystocia is a rare occurrence and an obstetric emergency. This occurs after the baby's head is delivered and the shoulders are too broad to be easily delivered. There are a series of maneuvers that your doctor will do. With your cooperation and the help of your partner in moving your legs, babies can be

safely delivered. If this occurs, time is of the essence, so please do as your doctor asks.

Cephalopelvic Disproportion (CPD)

Cephalopelvic disproportion means that the baby's head is too large to descend. Your doctor will do a cesarean section to deliver your baby.

THIRD STAGE OF LABOR: DELIVERY OF THE PLACENTA

This stage of labor lasts from five to thirty minutes. The placenta will usually deliver spontaneously. When the placenta has released from the uterus, your doctor will gently grasp the cord and ask you to push.

"Baby Shakes"

After delivery of the placenta, you may begin shaking. This can range from a mild shiver to uncontrollable shaking. The reason for this phenomenon is unclear, but it does happen. I call this "baby shakes."

Episiotomy/Laceration Repair

If you have had an episiotomy, your doctor will repair it after the placenta is delivered. A laceration can be a simple tear in the vaginal tissue or a complicated tear into the rectum (called a fourth-degree laceration). The latter must be repaired meticulously and takes some time. Your doctor will inform you if this has happened, and you will be asked to lie back so that the repair can be done easily. Each layer of tissue, from the rectum to the vagina, including the rectal sphincter muscle, is repaired layer by layer. A complication of a fourth-degree laceration is a rectovaginal fistula. This is a channel or track that extends from the vagina into the rectum. If you have had a fourth-degree laceration and pass stool through your vagina after you go home, you should notify your doctor.

COMPLICATIONS OF THIRD STAGE

Hemorrhage

Hemorrhage can occur before or after delivery of the placenta. If the uterus fails to contract after delivery, you can hemorrhage. This can be the result of overstretching the uterus with a large baby (macrosomia) or polyhydramnios. Infection, general anesthesia with halothane (a type of anesthetic gas) or retained placental tissue can also cause hemorrhage to occur. Other reasons for hemorrhage are deep lacerations of the vagina and cervix.

Placenta Accreta, Increta, Percreta

Placenta accreta means that the placenta has grown into the muscle fibers of the uterus. This is a rare condition. If only superficial attachment occurs (placenta accreta), the placenta may be removable. If the placenta grows halfway through the thickness of the muscle (placenta increta) or all the way through the muscle (placenta percreta), an emergency hysterectomy may be done.

Inversion of the Uterus

This is a literal turning inside out of the uterus. It is very rare but can be life threatening. The uterus must be placed into its proper position. Usually this can be done vaginally, but general anesthesia may be necessary. Sometimes this complication may require abdominal surgery to replace the uterus.

CESAREAN SECTION

Reasons

Cesarean section rates have increased dramatically in recent years. One of the biggest causes is repeat sections. The number of repeat cesarean sections should decrease as vaginal birth after cesarean becomes a norm everywhere.

There are other reasons for this type of delivery. Some do not become apparent until labor. Table 15–6 lists the absolute and relative reasons for cesarean delivery.

Table 15–6   Reasons for Cesarean Section

ABSOLUTE

Placenta previa	Prolapsed cord
Abruptio placentae	

RELATIVE
BEFORE LABOR

Macrosomia	Previous classical cesarean section
Rh iso-immunization	Postdate pregnancy
Abnormal presentation of fetus	Maternal health

DURING LABOR

Cephalopelvic disproportion	Arrest of labor
Fetal distress	Arrest of descent
Prolonged rupture of membranes	

Procedure

You and your doctor should discuss the reasons you may need a surgical delivery. Once the decision has been made, if there is not an emergency, you should receive epidural or spinal anesthesia. This will allow you to be awake and to see and touch your baby soon after birth. Your partner should be allowed to be with you in the operating room, unless an emergency situation is present.

You will be taken to the operating room and your anesthesia will be assessed. When you have adequate anesthesia, a foley catheter (a type of soft rubber tube) will be put into your bladder through the urethra.

There are two types of skin incisions that can be made: a vertical skin incision, which is a cut from your navel to the pubic bone, or a low, horizontal skin incision, also called a bikini incision, that goes just above or into your pubic hairline.

After the skin incision is made, all tissue layers are opened down to the uterus. Your bladder will be moved away from the uterus so that it is not injured. This can cause some sensitivity after the surgery. An incision will then be made in the uterus. There are two types of uterine incisions: classical (from the top of the uterus to the bottom) and low-transverse (a low incision above the cervix that goes across the uterus). The majority of uterine incisions are low-transverse. After the uterine incision is made, you will feel pressure applied to the top of your uterus as the baby's head is delivered. The baby's mouth and nose are suctioned free of mucus and fluid and the body delivered. The doctor will then clamp and cut the cord and hand the baby to the waiting pediatrician. After the baby is assessed and found to be healthy, your partner may hold the baby for you to see. You should talk to the baby and touch him.

The placenta will be removed. Closure of the uterus, replacing the bladder and closing all the layers of tissue in the abdominal wall are the next steps. Your skin may be closed with tiny stitches under the skin or with surgical staples that will be removed before you leave the hospital. You will be taken to a recovery room with your partner and baby, where you will remain for a period of time to allow the effects of anesthesia to wear off. You will then be taken to the postpartum room.

THE THERMOS BOTTLE

Michelle had pushed for three hours without progress. She and her husband, Thomas, had worked well together in labor. The baby, Zachary, was large and did not want to come out vaginally. After discussion, we decided to proceed with a cesarean section. Michelle was taken to the operating room while Thomas changed into a scrub suit. He sat at the head of the operating table beside his wife. After the baby was born, I held the baby over their heads above the surgical drape so they could see Zachary. I then handed the baby to the pediatrician. I informed Thomas that he could go to the infant warmer to see his son. He stated that he would stay where he was; he didn't want to see anything that was happening to Michelle.

The pediatrician assessed the baby and declared him healthy. The baby was then swaddled in a warm blanket, with his arms and legs tucked inside the blanket. A ski cap was placed on his head.

Zachary was now ready to meet his parents. The nurse took the baby to meet them. I heard a gasp from Thomas as he said, "My God, he looks like a thermos bottle! He doesn't have any arms or legs!" I then heard sobs coming from Michelle, as she asked if her baby was all right. I assured her that Zachary was fine. The nurse then proceeded to unwrap the baby so that they could see the arms and legs.

YOUR NEW BABY

What Baby Looks Like

If you have had a vaginal delivery, your baby may look like a wrinkled old man. The baby's head will be cone-shaped due to compression of the head as it passed through the pelvis and vagina.

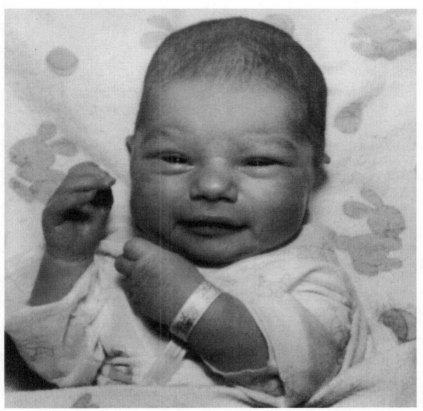

This cesarean baby was just as happy not to go through the birth canal.

This is called molding. The head will become round and normal-looking within a few days. If you have had a cesarean section, the baby may have a round head.

There are two soft spots called fontanelles on the baby's head. The larger, diamond-shaped one at the top of the baby's head will close by eighteen months of age. The much smaller, triangular one at the back of the head will close by six months of age.

The baby's eyelids will be puffy and the color of the eyes will most likely be blue. Its true eye color will develop by six months of age. The baby can see up to about eighteen inches away. The baby has received an antibiotic ointment in the eyes. This is done by law to protect newborns from gonorrhea.

The baby's shoulders and back may be covered with downy hair called lanugo. This will rub off in a few weeks. The baby may be bald, have a full head of hair or have something in between. Every baby is different.

The baby's skin will be blotchy and uneven in color. His hands and feet will have a bluish color and may be peeling. The baby may be covered with vernix. There may be marks on the baby's skin. The most common of these birthmarks are called stork bites, reddened blotches on the baby's face and neck. Stork bites disappear within a year. Other birthmarks are strawberry patches, which are red, raised marks that usually disappear; Mongolian spots, which are bruiselike marks on the lower backs of darkskinned babies that disappear; and port-wine stains, which are red to purple marks that do not disappear. Port-wine stains may require argon or other laser therapy if they are large or noticeable.

The baby's genitals will be swollen. This is the same for a boy or a girl and is the result of maternal hormones. The swelling will decrease in a few weeks.

The umbilical cord will be clamped close to the navel. It will dry and fall off within two weeks.

Your baby's appearance will change dramatically over the next few days.

Your baby's footprints are taken before you leave the delivery/birthing room. They will be on a certificate, along with your fingerprints. The certificate will have a number that matches the number on a bracelet that is put on the baby's wrist or ankle. You will have a matching bracelet. The numbers and footprints are for identification purposes.

What Baby Does

The baby will cry, sneeze, hiccup and make noises while breathing.

She will be unable to control her head to hold it upright; therefore you will need to support the baby's neck and head when you lift her or hold her.

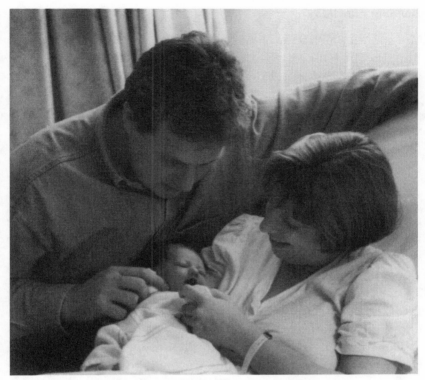

Take all the time you need to enjoy the wonder of your new baby.

Baby's senses are very acute at birth. She will bond to you by smell within a few days. Do not wear scented deodorant, perfume or aftershave lotion for several days after the baby is born. You want the baby to recognize *you* as her parents not Polo or White Diamonds.

If you have practiced fetal conditioning, your baby will seek out your voices. She will quiet to the sound of both of you. The music box will quiet and soothe her, especially if she cries inconsolably and nothing else works.

If touched on the cheek, your baby will turn in the direction of the touch and seek your breast. This is called the rooting reflex. The baby will make stepping movements if held upright with her feet touching a hard surface. When startled, she will throw out her arms and legs. This is called the Moro reflex.

Bonding with Baby

You should touch your baby, speak to him, cuddle him and caress him. Let the baby see your face as you talk. Speak in gentle tones. The baby will respond to your voice. Spend as much time as possible with your baby. Your baby will not be "spoiled" by too much holding. There is no such thing as too much bonding. The more you interact with your baby, the more connected to him you will feel.

To Circumcise or not to Circumcise: That Is the Question

Circumcision, the removal of part of the foreskin, has become a hotly debated topic recently. Fewer circumcisions are being done today. There is no medical reason, except rarely, for a circumcision, although some religions have made it part of their beliefs. The reason most circumcisions are done is cosmetic. The choice must be yours. You should research this as carefully as your choice of delivery method (see appendices).

The baby will be circumcised in the hospital when he is about twelve to twenty-four hours old. You may hold and soothe the baby during the procedure. Different methods are used today. One involves a metal bell-shaped instrument that is placed over the penis and clamped around the foreskin. The excess foreskin is removed with a scalpel. Another uses a clamplike device called a Mogan-Davey that is placed across the foreskin. The clamp is closed and the foreskin removed with a scalpel. You will be taught to care for the penis before you leave the hospital.

Complications for the Newborn

These conditions rarely occur and there is no need to worry that they will happen to your baby. However, you should be prepared for anything.

Infection

If mom develops a fever and uterine tenderness during labor, your baby may be infected also. This is called chorioamnionitis. The baby may be taken to the neonatal intensive care unit and have cultures of blood, urine and possibly spinal fluid taken. The baby may be placed on antibiotics until culture results are obtained. The most common cause of chorioamnionitis is B-strep bacteria. About 20 percent of all women can have B-strep in the vagina at any one time. This usually poses no problem and most babies will not get infected; however, some babies can become very ill. If the baby's cultures are positive for bacteria, she will receive seven to ten days of IV antibiotics.

Respiratory Distress Syndrome

Respiratory distress syndrome occurs primarily in premature babies and in babies of diabetic mothers. The baby is unable to breathe on its own because the lungs are immature. This can be fatal, but we now know a great deal about this complication. The use of infant respirators has changed the picture of this disease.

Meconium Aspiration

If your baby is stressed while still in the uterus, he can have a bowel movement. This first stool, called meconium, is dark and sticky. When mixed with the amniotic fluid, it can be aspirated by your baby during birth. If your amniotic fluid is meconium stained, your doctor will suction the baby thoroughly when the head is out and before the body is delivered. Pediatric attendants will be waiting to take the baby. They will intubate the baby and examine his vocal cords for meconium and meconium staining. If the baby has aspirated meconium, he will be taken to the intensive care unit, placed on oxygen, possibly intubated, and given IV antibiotics. The severity of the aspiration and how quickly the baby responds to treatment will determine the length of time the baby is in the unit.

Birth Injuries

Birth injuries are rare today, as the number of high- and mid-forceps deliveries has decreased.

Congenital Defects

Parents, nurses, doctors and midwives are upset when the baby has a congenital abnormality. Unsuspected congenital abnormalities are rare. These are so varied and can be so complicated that I will not discuss them specifically.

The baby will be taken to the intensive care unit, may have surgery soon after birth or may die.

The Intensive Care Unit

The special nursery for sick babies can be frightening. Your baby may be on a respirator and have an IV and monitoring equipment attached. Don't be afraid to touch and talk to your baby. The best medicine for your baby can be contact with loving parents. Visit the baby as much as possible.

IF A BABY DIES

No one likes to think about a baby dying, and the thought should not be there for you. However, if this tragedy happens, you need to know what to expect.

Stillborn

Modern obstetric techniques have dramatically decreased the number of babies that die before birth. Today almost every wanted pregnancy ends with the birth of a live, healthy baby.

Stillbirth accounts for more than half of perinatal deaths. The perinatal period is from twenty-eight weeks of gestation to six days after birth. The majority of fetal deaths occur between twenty-eight and thirty-two weeks. Approximately 30 percent are caused by asphyxia, which is lack of oxygen. Maternal complications, such as uncontrolled diabetes, hypertension, preeclampsia and abruptio placenta, cause approximately 25 percent. Congenital abnormalities account for approximately 20 percent. In 25 percent of fetal deaths, no reason can be found.

The diagnosis of fetal death is made by ultrasound. Most women who have a fetus die will go into spontaneous labor within two to three days. If you do not go into spontaneous labor, your doctor may induce labor. If you request delivery as soon as the diagnosis is made, your wish should be granted. You should be the one to decide if you want to be awake or sedated. The decision of where recovery will take place should also be yours.

During Labor

This is an extremely rare event. Use of modern obstetric techniques has almost eliminated this.

After Birth

The majority of babies that die after birth are premature. Postmaturity and congenital abnormalities are other causes.

Grieving

Mothers and fathers may show grief in very different ways, but both are grieving intensely. Everyone goes through the stages of grief (denial, bargaining, anger and guilt) differently before acceptance is achieved. You cannot deny grief; you must go through it, as exhausting and painful as it may be.

Some things may help. These include seeing and holding the baby as long and as often as you wish, having pictures taken of your baby and sharing your feelings with your partner. An autopsy may be helpful now and for future pregnancies. You may want to have burial services.

Always get grief counseling. This can be with an individual or in a support group. Consult the appendices for a resource list.

Most couples need at least six months to a year to grieve before another pregnancy should begin. You need to decide when the time is right for you to get pregnant again. Remember, every child is unique and special. One child can never replace another.

POSTPARTUM CARE

You have just worked extremely hard. Your hard work combined with a sudden decrease in pregnancy hormone levels will make you tired. Rest as much as possible. A good guide is to sleep when the baby does.

You will have uterine contractions after you deliver. These are called afterpains and will be more intense while breastfeeding because oxytocin, needed for milk letdown, causes uterine contractions. Afterpains usually go away after the first week to ten days. The uterus will begin involution, decreasing to its prepregnancy size.

The bleeding and discharge you have after delivery is called lochia. Your lochia will be red for several days, then change to a brown color. This will eventually change to yellow and decrease in amount. You should use hospital sanitary pads the first few days because they are more comfortable.

Your perineum has been stretched and will be sore for many days. Use an ice pack for the first twenty-four hours after delivery. Sitz baths may also help relieve the soreness. Always clean yourself from front to back to avoid infections. After urination, wash the perineum with a spray bottle called a peribottle. Witch hazel may be very helpful to use. Soak a cotton ball with witch hazel and blot the perineum. You can start your Kegel exercises as soon as the soreness lessens.

If you have had an episiotomy, you must care for it meticulously, following the same suggestions given for the perineum. Sitz baths are especially helpful in relieving soreness. Avoid bending your knees to pick up objects, as this may add stress to the episiotomy.

If you have hemorrhoids, they may be swollen and inflamed after pushing. There are several suggestions that may help. Use witch hazel after each bowel movement. Eat a high-fiber diet, drink plenty of fluids and, if your stool is still too hard, ask your doctor to prescribe a stool softener. If you have had an episiotomy, hold tissue against it as you bear down.

Urination may be uncomfortable due to swelling. Drink plenty of fluids and relax. Do not strain to urinate, as this will cause more swelling.

Showers are recommended until your lochia is yellow.

Breastfeeding will require care of the breasts. Keep them clean. You may need to massage nipples with vitamin E oil if they become dry or cracked. Be sure to wash the vitamin E oil off before feeding the baby. Wear a good nursing bra. If you are not breastfeeding, wear a tight bra all the time, even when sleeping.

Eat what you want to eat, but continue to follow a healthy diet.

Postoperative Care

In addition to the recommendations given for a vaginal delivery, you should follow specific recommendations for after surgery.

You will be very tired, you have worked hard, your hormones have suddenly decreased and you have had major surgery. Rest as much as possible.

You will have a catheter in your bladder and an IV that will keep you hydrated. You will be kept in bed for at least twelve hours after the c-section. The bladder catheter will be removed when you are permitted to get out of bed. You should always have help the first few times you get out of bed.

Clear liquids should be allowed almost as soon as your section is finished. As soon as you can tolerate it, you will be given a regular diet. This is usually one or two days after the surgery. The IV will be taken out when you can drink liquids without a problem.

Increase your activity gradually over several days. Most patients are able to walk without help by the third day.

Pain medications will be given either by IV or by injection the first day. After this, you should be able to take medication orally. Most patients do not require strong pain medication by the third day.

Bowel movements may be slow to resume. This can be the result of the pain medications and the open abdomen during surgery.

Your incision should be kept clean and dry.

You may have shoulder pain after surgery as a result of air or blood irritating your diaphragm. This will decrease in about a day.

Breastfeeding may be uncomfortable due to the incision and the difficulty you have in getting around. Take your time and find a comfortable position for you, then feed.

CHAPTER SIXTEEN

CUTTING THE APRON STRINGS

Going Home

LEAVING THE HOSPITAL

Rooming in, having the baby with you at all times and allowing fathers to stay overnight have done a great deal to take the fear out of going home with a new baby. Staying as a family unit after birth allows bonding.

You absolutely *must* have a safety car seat to take the baby home.

You will sign an identification document with the numbers given at birth to verify that the baby is yours. If you have had an uncomplicated vaginal delivery, you may go home in twenty-four hours; you will rest better at home in your own surroundings. A c-section requires a few more days in the hospital. In this case, you may go home three days after delivery.

Your prepregnancy clothes will not fit immediately after delivery, so don't expect them to. Wear comfortable, loose-fitting clothes.

If you have other children, have them come to the hospital to see the new baby and, if possible, help to take you home. If they cannot visit, a special welcome home surprise for you and the new baby should be planned by them.

VISITORS

Everyone wants to see the new baby; however, you need rest, time with your partner, time with your new baby, time with your other children and time for yourself. Being a hostess can be exhausting.

You do not need to do this the first few weeks at home. Suggest that visitors not come for two weeks. If you need to blame someone for not having visitors, blame it on your doctor. Put a message on your answering machine telling people that the baby has arrived and that you will return their calls after you have rested. You need time to adjust to your new, permanent houseguest, and she needs time to adjust and become part of the family.

MOMMY CARE

AFTER VAGINAL DELIVERY

REST
You will need a great deal of rest the first few weeks after delivery. The delivery, the increased demands of the baby and the interruption in your sleep will make you tired. You should rest when the baby sleeps.

EXERCISE
Exercise will actually help decrease fatigue, as well as increase your muscle tone and energy level.

You may begin exercising as soon as you feel ready. Pelvic tilts, modified situps, hip walking, stretches and other abdominal exercises are excellent. There are numerous books and videos available that will show the correct way to do postpartum exercises (see appendices).

DIET
You should lose up to twenty pounds the first two weeks after delivery. If you maintain your healthy prepregnancy diet, you should lose the rest of your baby weight by six to eight weeks after delivery.

If you're breastfeeding, you will need to increase your pregnancy diet by 300 calories a day. You also need extra fluids, calcium and protein. You should avoid spicy foods, alcohol, nicotine and drugs while breastfeeding, since these can be passed on to your baby through your breast milk.

BREAST CARE

Colostrum will be made the first two or three days after delivery. Engorgement of the breasts occurs two to four days after delivery due to milk letdown. If you experience pain, ice packs applied to the breasts four or five times a day and acetaminophen may help.

BOTTLE FEEDING

Your doctor may give you medication to keep your milk from coming in; however, other measures may work equally well. Discuss side effects of the medication with your doctor before taking it. Do not express milk if you have letdown. This will just encourage more milk production. Binding your breasts and using ice will help. Tightly wrap a cloth approximately ten to twelve inches wide around your chest two or three times. You should rewrap every few hours and sleep with the wrapping in place. Continue wrapping for five to seven days. Avoid bending over. After wrapping, wear a good supportive bra. If you wear your bra twenty-four hours a day for the first few weeks after delivery, your breasts should not sag.

BREASTFEEDING

Wear a good supportive nursing bra. Keep nipples clean and soft. If nipples become dry and cracked, use vitamin E oil to soften them. Be sure to wash and dry nipples before breastfeeding if you use vitamin E oil or lotion. Breasts do leak, and this can be embarrassing. Using disposable breast pads inside your bra will keep your clothing from being stained and may decrease your chances of having dry, cracked breasts. If you wear a good supportive bra, your breasts will not sag and will return to prepregnancy size. If you have breast implants, check with your doctor to see if you should breastfeed. It is not recommended that you breastfeed if you have silicone implants; however, this could change, and your doctor will recommend what is best for you and your baby.

A breast infection, called mastitis, is common. The bacteria that cause the infection come from the baby's mouth. The breast will be painful, hot and swollen and you may run a fever. If you develop an infection, your doctor will prescribe antibiotics. You can continue to breastfeed while taking the antibiotics.

PERINEAL CARE

If you have had an episiotomy or a tear, you may find that it is difficult to sit on hard surfaces. Carry a soft pillow with you. It may make it easier to sit.

Continue the same episiotomy and perineal care you began in the hospital. After showers, use a blow dryer on a low setting instead of a towel to dry the perineal area. Continue until your episiotomy is well healed.

AFTER CESAREAN SECTION

REST

You will require more rest for a longer period of time after a c-section. Gradually increase your activity to a normal level over several weeks. Avoid heavy lifting and going up and down stairs.

INCISION CARE

Keep the incision clean and dry. Avoid heavy lifting and stretching.

DIET

For the first few weeks, follow the same diet you followed while pregnant. You should then eliminate the extra 300 calories a day that you added to your normal, healthy diet.

EXERCISE

You should not exercise until your doctor has given permission.

PHYSICAL CHANGES

Your body will undergo many physical and hormonal changes during the first few weeks after delivery.

UTERUS

Involution of the uterus will continue for several weeks. By the end of the second week your uterus will be about the size of a twelve-week pregnancy. Five to six weeks after delivery, it will be almost prepregnancy size.

CERVIX

The cervix will close and become firm by the time the uterus involutes to prepregnancy size.

VAGINA

Your vagina was stretched during the vaginal delivery, but it should regain its muscle tone by six weeks postpartum. You can accelerate the process and increase muscle tone by doing Kegel exercises. Kegel exercises, which tighten and relax your pelvic floor muscles, use the same muscles that you utilize to stop a flow of urine or have a bowel movement. Tighten by thinking of stopping urine flow or stopping a bowel movement. Begin with five repetitions three times a day. Increase by one or two repetitions a day until you are doing twenty-five repetitions three times a day. You can begin Kegel exercises twenty-four hours after delivery.

HORMONAL CHANGES

Progesterone and estrogen levels fall dramatically in the first seventy-two hours after delivery. Progesterone decreases to 1/20th of the pregnancy levels and estrogen decreases to 1/100th of the pregnancy levels. These changes remain in effect until ovulation occurs.

RETURN OF MENSTRUATION

Ovulation can return as early as four weeks after delivery in a woman who is not breastfeeding, but it can be as long as twelve weeks.

In breastfeeding women, it can take as long as thirty-six months for ovulation to return if breastfeeding is continued the entire time.

Ovulation precedes a period, so you must use birth control with sex. Up to 5 percent of breastfeeding women will ovulate the first six months; you cannot be sure you aren't one of them.

CIRCULATION

Your blood volume, which increased by 35 percent during pregnancy, will begin decreasing rapidly immediately after delivery, then slow until prepregnancy levels are reached by six weeks postpartum. Some of this decrease will result from delivery. The balance of excess fluid will be eliminated by the kidneys. You will notice an increase in urination and sweating after delivery.

ABDOMEN

Abdominal muscles have been stretched throughout the pregnancy. It will take time and work to get them back to prepregnancy control and tone. You can begin abdominal exercises twenty-four hours after a vaginal delivery, but if you have had a c-section, wait until your doctor advises you when to begin.

SKIN

Skin changes will gradually return to normal. Stretch marks fade to a silvery color by six months to a year after birth. The linea nigra will fade but will always be darker than before pregnancy.

EMOTIONAL CHANGES

Your emotions and mental processes are profoundly affected during the first few weeks after delivery. Although the sudden drop in hormone levels is usually blamed, research has not supported this theory. There may, however, be a relationship between low levels of tryptophan, an amino acid, and the emotional changes seen after delivery. Sleep deprivation and increased work caused by demands of the baby may also contribute.

"BABY BLUES"

Up to 70 percent of women will have "baby blues." The symptoms include crying for no apparent reason; depression; sudden mood swings, headaches, restlessness, irritability, confusion, forgetfulness, insomnia feelings of resentment toward the baby and/or your partner and elation. You probably will not have all of the symptoms. "Baby blues" can happen any time during the first two weeks after delivery and may last for a week. Support from those around you, adequate rest and good nutrition may all help. "Baby blues" are so common that if you don't get them, you're lucky. Know that you're normal and they'll go away.

POSTPARTUM DEPRESSION

Approximately 10 percent of new mothers will develop postpartum depression. This can be a serious medical problem that requires intervention by your doctor. The symptoms are the same as for "baby blues" but also include a loss of self-esteem; a sense of hopelessness; an inability to care for yourself, your family or the baby; and negative feelings toward your baby.

With medication, you should be better in a few weeks. Family support is essential. You need adequate rest and help in caring for your family. They need to understand what is happening to you.

POSTPARTUM PSYCHOSIS

This is a very rare schizophrenic and manic-depressive disorder that can happen in approximately 1 in 1,000 women. Most women recover in two or three months with medication and psychiatric intervention.

COMPLICATIONS THAT CAN OCCUR

In addition to postpartum depression, possible complications include uterine infection; bladder infection; thrombophlebitis, or a blood clot in a vessel; breast infection; retained fragments of placenta; infection in the episiotomy; and infection in the abdominal incision.

When to Call Your Doctor

Contact your doctor if you develop a fever; if you notice bright red bleeding after your lochia has changed to brown or yellow; if you notice redness, tenderness or a hot lump in your breast; if you develop a foul-smelling vaginal discharge; if you notice increased pain in your episiotomy; if you notice a drainage or redness in your abdominal incision; or if you are depressed and exhibit loss of appetite, extreme mood swings, uncontrollable crying and feelings that you want to hurt your baby.

DADDY CARE

EMOTIONAL CHANGES

You have bonded with your baby before birth, but you may not be prepared for the depth of attachment and love you have for this child. You may become preoccupied while at work with thoughts of the new baby and mom. You will miss them when you are away. At the same time, you may resent the child because of the drastic changes that have happened in your life.

Babies are slave drivers. They demand attention and many times will not wait until you are able to give it. You may wonder how something so small can create so much work. There seems to be an endless list of things to do. If you've returned to work, you may feel even more overwhelmed. Add to this the lack of sleep the first several weeks. Your other children may also be demanding more time from you. If you think of all the sudden changes in your life, you will understand how you can love your new baby and possibly resent him at the same time.

DON'T FORGET THE BABY

Amy and Kurt came in for the six-week checkup carrying a ten-pound bundle of smiles named Sarah. They were delighted with their daughter. After Amy's examination, I sat holding the baby and asked how things were going. Amy and Kurt looked at each other and burst out laughing. I was reminded that I had told them not to forget the baby the first time they went out. At that time, they assured me that it was the silliest thing they had ever heard. They then told me about the first time they went to visit Grandma with the baby. After an hour of preparation, getting all the baby things in order and packed in the car, they were ready to leave. They went over the list of things they had packed to make sure they hadn't forgotten anything. Positive that everything was in the car, they left the house and were locking the door when Amy suddenly shrieked, "We forgot the baby!" Sarah was sound asleep in her crib.

You may find that sex is almost nonexistent for many weeks or months following the birth of the baby. This can be the result of many things besides the physical trauma of childbirth to your partner's body. Basically you may both be too tired or just not in the mood.

You may sometimes be overwhelmed by what you don't know about parenting. This is a normal feeling. No one expects you to have all the answers. Men do not have the emotional support in our society for the new father role. Just as you need to be a part of the family, you also need to have friends. Sometimes you may feel forgotten, as everyone gives attention to the new baby and mom. Relax and use the time to enjoy the role of father.

You need time alone with your new baby, a time when you can cuddle, talk to and play. Take the time you need to spend with your child.

Time with your partner is also important. The demands of parenthood can cause stress in your relationship. You need time together to heal that.

Continue to spend time as a family as you did before the baby was born. Remember, being a parent can bring great joy.

BIG BROTHER/SISTER CARE

Spend time alone with your older child. This may be difficult at times, especially when you're tired. Let your child know that you love him and that he is still special to you. As always, though, disruptive behavior should be corrected. Provide new activities or games. While you're interacting with the new baby, discuss big brother with the new baby. Your child will hear this and feel that he has a special place in the baby's life.

If your older child wishes to help with the baby, allow him to get diapers and other supplies for you, or talk or sing to the baby when you bathe, change or feed her. Even a very young child will feel part of the activity if he is given something to do. The older child may feel left out as visitors come to see the new baby and bring gifts. Let him open the gifts for the baby, if he is old enough. If your older child does not want to interact with the new baby, respect his wishes. He will see that you are not forcing him and will soon become interested.

PET CARE

Your pet has been a part of your family. Remember, it's used to all your attention if this is your first baby. You must treat it as though it were an older sibling, in the sense that you want to pay attention to it and not create an atmosphere of jealousy.

If possible, bring home an item of clothing the baby has worn at the hospital. Allow your pet to smell the baby's scent.

Pets are curious. Let your pet smell the baby and see her when you come home from the hospital. Your pet may want to see what you do with the baby.

Small dogs will sometimes treat a baby as their puppy and be fiercely protective. Large dogs can also be fiercely protective.

Cats cannot, as the old wives' tale says, "steal the baby's breath," nor do they smother babies.

Animals do carry different bacteria and diseases than humans, so keep face-to-face contact to a minimum.

LIVING SPACE CARE

Your apartment or house will not fall apart if you do not personally take care of it. You should have help the first two weeks you are home. If you have had a c-section, you may wish to have help for longer than two weeks. Your help can be friends, relatives or hired help, such as the child care person you have engaged or a doula, a woman who cares for you and your house while you care for your baby. Your help should take care of you, your partner, other children, if you have them, and the living space. You and your partner need time with your new baby, to bond and get to know her.

BABY CARE: YOUR BABY'S FIRST SIX WEEKS

Whether breast or bottle feeding, this is an excellent time to interact with your baby. Sing or talk to her in a soothing tone of voice. Look at her and make eye contact. Your baby can see you very clearly.

Bottle Feeding

If you have decided to bottle feed, you should get your pediatrician's recommendations on which formula to use. You can purchase most formulas in ready-to-feed or concentrated form. Check to see which type of concentration you have.

Preparation and Sterilization

Bottles can be prepared either by adding the formula and then sterilizing or by sterilizing the bottles, then pouring in the formula. To prepare bottles with the formula inside, first wash bottles, nipples, disks, rings and covers thoroughly. Pour the amount of formula needed into each bottle. If concentrated formula is used, first add the correct amount of water. After filling the bottles, invert the nipples inside the bottle and place the disk and ring on loosely. Put the filled bottles in a sterilizer with three to four inches of water. Bring to a boil, cover sterilizer and boil for twenty-five minutes. When finished boiling, tighten rings and put on cap.

To prepare bottles first, wash bottles, nipples, caps, disks and rings thoroughly. Place the bottles upside down in the sterilizer and add the other bottle parts. Add five to six inches of water and boil for five minutes. Fill the bottles with prepared formula, invert nipple to inside, place disk and ring, tighten and cap.

All prepared bottles should be stored in the refrigerator. Do not reuse formula that has been at room temperature for more than an hour. Do not use a microwave to heat a bottle. Instead, heat a bottle using a saucepan with boiling water. Always test the temperature on the inside of your wrist to make sure the formula is not too hot. Burp your baby after every two ounces of formula.

Breastfeeding

The baby should feed on demand the first few weeks. This will prevent breast engorgement and give the baby the maximum amount of milk possible the crucial first few weeks. After the first weeks, your baby should settle down to a routine and not feed as often.

The secrets to successful breastfeeding are maternal relaxation and proper latching on to the breast. Touch the baby's cheek so that she turns toward the breast. Her mouth will open instinctively. Direct the nipple into the baby's open mouth by grasping your breast and guiding it. When correctly latched on, the baby's mouth will be on breast tissue, not your nipple. Her tongue and jaw will work to suck the milk.

Allow the baby to nurse from the first breast as long as she likes, then switch to the other breast. At the next feeding begin with the breast used last in the previous feeding.

To break the suction established between the baby and the breast, gently insert your finger into the baby's mouth.

Positions for breastfeeding can vary and are dependent on comfort. You can hold your baby under your arm, like a football, and resting on a pillow. Feed her from the same side you're holding her. Another position is lying on your side with the baby next to you. These are both good positions if you have had a c-section. The baby held in both arms, head held higher than her body with her stomach against yours, is the most comfortable position once the baby learns to feed properly.

Breast milk can be pumped and stored to use if you're not home when the baby needs to be fed. Be sure that the bottle does not have cross-cut nipples, since these can change the baby's sucking pattern. Breast milk can be refrigerated for forty-eight hours and frozen for up to six months.

Sleeping

All babies are different. Some are quiet and sleep more often and for longer periods. Others are more active and sleep less often and for shorter periods. How often your baby sleeps will depend on how often he eats. Babies do not have a routine pattern until three to six weeks of age. Babies can start sleeping through the night as early as three months of age.

Newborn babies sleep twelve to twenty hours a day. They can be in a light sleep state in which they are easily aroused. Their breathing is irregular and they smile, move, cry or suck. Some babies stay at this level of sleep for several weeks after birth. Others fall from this into a deeper sleep state.

In a deep sleep, babies have regular breathing and do not arouse easily. If aroused, they will go back to sleep. Babies may make sudden, jerking movements while in a deep sleep.

Time Awake

When your baby awakens from sleep, he may be drowsy. His breathing will be irregular and he may either return to sleep or become alert.

Your baby can be quietly or actively alert. Quiet alertness is a calm period in which the baby focuses on what he sees or hears. This is the best time to elicit a response when you talk, sing or play with your baby.

Fatigue, hunger, noises, excessive handling and wet diapers can affect your baby's mood when he is actively alert. Your baby will fuss and cry. Feed him, change his diaper and comfort him quickly so that he may return to calmness. If you do not act quick enough to suit him, the baby will continue crying.

Crying is the way your baby communicates his needs. Sometimes, however, a baby will cry for no apparent reason. If you have attended to all his needs and comforting doesn't help, playing his music box may calm and soothe him. If this doesn't work, try wrapping him snugly, rocking him, laying him on a lambskin, taking him for a ride, turning on a household appliance that makes a low humming noise, such as a dishwasher, or giving him a pacifier. Crying exercises the lungs and is a necessary function. Don't panic if the baby cries "just because."

Crying and drawing his legs up may signal that your baby has colic. No one knows why babies are colicky. If your baby is colicky, trying various comfort techniques may help. These include offering him a pacifier; walking him; rocking him; going for a car ride; using a device under the crib mattress or on the crib rail that gently rocks the mattress; wrapping him snugly; holding him against your skin for warmth; placing a warm water bottle

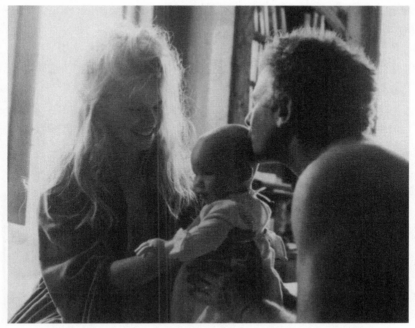

By six weeks of age, the baby is comfortable and interactive with Mom and Dad and his environment.

wrapped in a towel or blanket against his abdomen; putting him in a front carrier facing you; and giving him very, very weak camomile tea or peppermint water. Peppermint soothes stomach and gas pain. Put a peppermint Lifesaver in a bottle with four ounces of warm water. Shake for five seconds and remove the Lifesaver.

You can never give your baby too much attention or spoil him by holding him too much. Babies love attention and love being held. There is no such thing as too much love.

Milestones

From birth, your baby will begin to do things and reveal her personality. Table 16–1 lists the most common developmental milestones from birth to six weeks of age. Remember, though, that your baby is an individual and will do things at her own pace. If your baby was premature, these milestones may be delayed.

TABLE 16–1   *Developmental Milestones—Birth to Six Weeks*

What Baby Does	Age
Turns toward sound and pays attention to it	Birth to six weeks
Controls head for a few moments	Birth to four weeks
Follows an object with her eyes	Birth to six weeks
Looks at your face	Birth to four weeks
Smiles when you talk to her	Three weeks to two months
Holds head up when lying on stomach	Five weeks to three months
Holds head steady	Six weeks to four months
Laughs	Six weeks to four months

Bathing

You should sponge bathe the baby until her umbilical cord falls off. Gently wash her head daily.

You should begin to put the baby in water as soon as possible after the cord falls off. Use a baby bathtub, basin or sink, and make sure the water is warm, not hot. Use your elbow or wrist to test the temperature. Keep all baby bath supplies and clothing close at hand. You may want to cut the baby's nails now using blunt baby scissors. Wash your baby's face first with either plain water or, as she gets older, a mild baby soap. Gently place the baby into the water feet first, and using your hand, put water over her body. Babies love water. Use a mild baby soap and be sure to rinse the baby well. Place your arm under her shoulder and grasp around the other armpit; in this way, she will not slip out of your grasp. You should wash her head last. Your baby loses heat quickly from her head and you don't want her to become chilled. After bathing, wrap the baby with a towel and place her on a flat surface. Quickly towel dry. You may want to do baby exercises at this time or simply dress the baby. Never leave your baby alone in the water.

UMBILICAL CORD CARE
The baby's umbilical cord will fall off usually within two weeks. You should apply alcohol to it every time you change the baby. This will help the cord to dry. Do not pull at it or try to force it to come off. Make sure the top of the diaper is folded underneath the cord. Some newborn disposable diapers feature a cutout at the top that will accommodate the umbilical cord.

CIRCUMCISION CARE
If your baby boy has had a circumcision, the penis needs to be kept clean using a wet cotton ball. Then apply a liberal amount of an antibiotic ointment until the penis has healed completely. This routine should be done with each diaper change. Using an antibiotic ointment will reduce the risk of infection and keep the diaper from sticking to the penis.

UNCIRCUMCISED CARE
Bathe your baby normally, cleaning the penis gently. DO NOT TRY TO RETRACT THE FORESKIN. It is attached and will become fully retractable on its own by age three to five.

Clothing

Your baby is not aware of fashion yet, just comfort. Clothes should be soft and loose. Babies move around a great deal; therefore, they should not be put in restrictive clothing. Clothing should not have decorations that could come off. The layette list in the appendices can give you ideas on what baby should wear. Do not buy extra articles now that the baby has arrived. You will find that your baby will quickly grow out of clothes.

Bowel Movements and Urination

Your baby will urinate often during the day and night. Be sure to notice if there is a decrease in the frequency of urination.

Bowel movements depend on how you are feeding your baby. Stools for bottle-fed babies are firmer, darker and less frequent than for breastfed babies. Breastfed babies have frequent, loose stools that vary from pastelike to liquid with curds. The color varies from light yellow to a light brown. It is not unusual for the baby to have a bowel movement after each feeding.

Diapers

Cloth diapers or disposable diapers—the choice is yours. Disposable diapers are convenient but can be expensive. You should use environmentally friendly disposable diapers, if this is your choice.

Cloth diapers can be a chore since you need a place to store soiled ones before washing. A diaper service may be the answer.

Well-Baby Care

Your baby should see her pediatrician for her first well-baby visit during the first six weeks. The baby will be weighed and measured, and her eyes, ears, nose, mouth, heart, lungs and abdomen will be assessed. If you have any questions, ask the doctor at this first visit.

Illness

Mild jaundice, a yellow tint to the baby's skin, can be found in half of all newborns. It is caused by bilirubin, which forms when the red blood cells break down. Bilirubin is then processed by the liver. However, newborn livers do not work efficiently until one to two years of age. Jaundice first appears after two or three days and disappears by two weeks of age. If the jaundice is significant, it can signal other problems. These can include Rh incompatibility; blood-type incompatibility; and reactions to drugs used during labor, such as pitocin. You should notify your pediatrician if you suspect jaundice. Your doctor will do a blood test to determine the level of bilirubin and, if it is high, may treat the baby with phototherapy, placing the baby under lights.

Your baby may cry when she doesn't feel well. Signs of illness in babies can be lethargy, loss of appetite, fever, vomiting, watery diarrhea and listless inattention. Talk to your pediatrician. He or she will help you learn when these things are signs of illness and when they are not.

If the baby exhibits forceful, projectile vomiting, notify your pediatrician at once. This may signal a serious medical condition.

When to Call the Pediatrician

Contact your doctor if the baby has watery diarrhea, is vomiting forcefully, will not eat, is lethargic, has a fever or is listlessly inattentive.

GRANDPARENT CARE

Some grandparents may seem reluctant at first because they do not wish to interfere. Others may overwhelm you with advice. Listen politely, thank them, then remember that this is your baby and you can do things the way you want. If grandparents are coming to help with the new baby, set a date beforehand for their departure. They only have your best interest at heart, of course, but they can sometimes be overwhelming, and this can lead to more stress for all of you.

THREE-WEEK CHECKUP

Exam

Not all practitioners have new mothers return for a three-week checkup. If you have a three-week checkup, your perineum should be examined if you have had a vaginal delivery or your incision examined if you have had a c-section.

Sex

Discuss this with your doctor at this visit. Usually, you may resume sex when it is comfortable for you. Use a condom to prevent infection if you resume intercourse during the first six weeks after the baby is born. The first few times may be a little uncomfortable. Make sure you are well lubricated and ask your partner to be very gentle. This should be enjoyable for both of you. Some women are ready to resume sex in three weeks, others in three months. You should do what is comfortable for you. Discuss with your partner your desires.

Birth Control

Birth control options should be discussed at this visit to give you time to make a choice before your six-week exam. The birth control options available today are listed in Table 16–2.

SIX-WEEK CHECKUP

Examination

At your postpartum examination, you should have your weight, blood pressure, breasts and abdomen assessed. A pelvic examination should include a Pap smear and assessment of whether your reproductive system has returned to normal.

You should discuss the method of birth control you have cho-

TABLE 16-2   Contraceptive Guide

Discuss the risks and benefits of each method with your doctor and along with that adivce, select the most suitable method for you as a couple.

Method	How It Works	Advantages	Disadvantages	How to Use It
THE PILL	Man-made hormones (estrogen and progesterone) similar to the ones your body naturally produces monthly, prevent the egg from maturing and being released from the ovary. No egg—no pregnancy. The pill also causes changes in the lining of the uterus and in the consistency of the cervical mucus. EFFECTIVENESS: 99% AVERAGE	Reduces the risk of ovarian cancer, uterine cancer, pelvic inflammatory disease. May decrease menstrual cramps and bleeding. Periods are more regular. Return to fertility immediate upon stopping pill. Does not interfere with lovemaking.	Not safe for everyone. Needs prescription, must be taken daily. Cannot be used by those with history of breast cancer, blood clots or at risk to develop blood clots, unexplained uterine bleeding, smokers over age 35, those on the drug Rifampin. Probably should not be used by those with light periods, high blood pressure, diabetes, migraine headaches,	A hormone pill is taken for 21 days, then no pill or a sugar pill is taken for 7 days to complete a 28-day cycle.

TABLE 16-2   Contraceptive Guide (cont.)

Method	How It Works	Advantages	Disadvantages	How to Use It
THE PILL (cont.)	COST: $20–$25/MONTH		depression, sickle cell trait, fibroids. A small percentage of users can develop serious side effects including: blood clots, liver disease, high blood pressure, gall bladder disease, migraine headaches. Less serious side effects include: nausea, breast tenderness (although the pill helps this in some women), mid-cycle bleeding for the first few months, weight gain, mood swings, depression, headaches. May need to use barrier method	

TABLE 16-2   Contraceptive Guide *(cont.)*

Method	How It Works	Advantages	Disadvantages	How to Use It
THE PILL *(cont.)*			if pill missed or antibiotics taken. One can forget to take pill.	
IMPLANTS	Small tubes containing progesterone, similar to what your body produces, slowly release small amounts of the hormone preventing release of eggs from the ovaries. No egg—no pregnancy. Also causes changes in the lining of the uterus and cervical mucus.	Works up to five years or until removed. Fertility returns immediately upon removal of implants. Helps protect against uterine cancer. Can be used safely after childbirth and while breastfeeding. Does not interfere with lovemaking.	Requires a minor surgical procedure to place and remove. Cannot be used by women with liver disease, breast cancer, unexplained uterine bleeding, blood clots. May not be good for women with high blood pressure, gall bladder disease, elevated cholesterol, irregular periods, light periods, headaches, heart disease. Side	Six match-sized tubes containing progesterone are placed surgically under the skin in the upper arm.

TABLE 16-2 *Contraceptive Guide (cont.)*

Method	How It Works	Advantages	Disadvantages	How to Use It
IMPLANTS (*cont.*)	EFFECTIVENESS: 99%+ AVERAGE COST: $450–$750/5 years		effects can include: irregular bleeding, prolonged periods, light periods, hair loss, decreased interest in sex. Some implants can be seen and felt.	Must get injection every three months.
INJECTIONS	An injection containing a hormone, progesterone, similar to what your body produces, prevents release of the egg from the ovary. It also causes changes in cervical mucus and the lining of the uterus.	Highly effective, helps protect against uterine cancer, safe after childbirth and while breastfeeding. Does not interfere with lovemaking. One injection every 3 months.	Must be given by a health care professional, prescription needed. Long-acting, fertility returns 6–18 months after the last injection. Should not be used if pregnancy is desired within the year. Should not be used by women with: blood clots, breast	

TABLE 16-2   *Contraceptive Guide (cont.)*

Method	How It Works	Advantages	Disadvantages	How to Use It
INJECTIONS (*cont.*)	EFFECTIVENESS: 99%+ AVERAGE COST: $25–$50 EVERY 3 MONTHS		cancer, liver disease, unexplained uterine bleeding. May not be good for women with family history of breast cancer, abnormal mammogram, irregular or light periods, high blood pressure, migraine headaches, asthma, epilepsy, diabetes, depression. Side effects can include: irregular periods, loss of interest in sex, bloating/weight gain, headaches, depression, possible mineral bone loss.	

TABLE 16-2   Contraceptive Guide (cont.)

Method	How It Works	Advantages	Disadvantages	How to Use It
IUD	Two types are available: a progesterone impregnated IUD and a copper T-shaped IUD. The IUD may prevent pregnancy by interfering with sperm movement, the ability of the sperm to fertilize the egg or interfere with the implantation or nesting of a fertilized egg into the lining of the uterus. EFFECTIVENESS: CopperT: 99%; Progesterone	Requires no attention except for monthly checks for the string. Fertility returns immediately upon removal. Does not interfere with lovemaking. Copper IUD needs to be changed only every eight years; the progesterone IUD must be changed yearly.	Requires a health care professional to place and remove it. Should not be used by women who have never had children, still want children, have multiple sex partners, or have a history of pelvic inflammatory disease or tubal pregnancy. Side effects may include: cramps, backache, spotting, heavy periods. May have an increased risk for tubal pregnancy, pelvic inflammatory disease, infertility. May be	A health care practitioner inserts the IUD, usually at the time of a period. You must check the string after every period.

TABLE 16-2   Contraceptive Guide (*cont.*)

Method	How It Works	Advantages	Disadvantages	How to Use It
IUD (*cont.*)	IUD: 97%. AVERAGE COST: CopperT $200–$400/8 years; progesterone IUD $200–$300/year.		expelled without knowing it.	
SPERMICIDES *Foams, creams, vaginal inserts*	Forms a chemical barrier that kills the sperm or makes sperm inactive and thus unable to pass through the cervix to the egg. No sperm— no pregnancy. EFFECTIVENESS: 80% AVERAGE COST: $0.50–$3.00 per use.	Available without a prescription. No known risks to general health. Fertility returns immediately upon discontinued use.	Less effective than other methods. Effectiveness can be increased if used with condoms. Side effects: Vaginal irritation, some women allergic to spermicides. May interrupt lovemaking. Only last for one sex act.	Must be applied into the vagina within 30 minutes of ejaculation. Inserts may need to be placed one hour before intercourse. Must follow package instructions.

TABLE 16-2   *Contraceptive Guide (cont.)*

Method	How It Works	Advantages	Disadvantages	How to Use It
DIAPHRAGM	A rubber dome that forms a barrier to prevent sperm from reaching the cervix. Spermicide, which is always used with it, kills or immobilizes sperm. EFFECTIVENESS: 85% AVERAGE COST: $15–$40 per diaphragm plus the cost of spermicide.	Can be inserted up to two hours before lovemaking. Safe. Fertility returns immediately with discontinued use.	Must be fitted by a health care professional and needs prescription. Must be used each time. Spermicides must be added with each new act without removing the diaphragm. May have an increase in urinary tract infections. Some women are allergic to spermicides. May need to be refitted after a 10 pound weight change, pregnancy. Must be replaced periodically. Must be left in place 6–8 hours. May decrease spontaneity.	Apply spermicide and place diaphragm deep into the vagina, over the cervix.

TABLE 16-2   Contraceptive Guide (*cont.*)

Method	How It Works	Advantages	Disadvantages	How to Use It
CERVICAL CAP	Rubber/plastic dome or cap that fits tightly over the cervix. Should be used with spermicide to place it, which kills sperm. Held in place by suction. EFFECTIVENESS: 85% AVERAGE COST: $25–$50 per cap	May be left in place 24–48 hours. Less spermicide is used than the diaphragm. No need to apply more spermicide with each act of intercourse. Fertility returns immediately with discontinued use.	Must be fitted by a health care professional. May become dislodged. Must be left in place 8 hours after intercourse.	Spermicide is placed in the cap which is then placed snugly over the cervix.
SPONGE	A soft, polyurethane sponge saturated with spermicide blocks and kills or immobilizes the sperm.	Needs no prescription. Safe for general health. Can be inserted any time and left in place up to 24 hours with multiple acts of	Needs to be left in place 6 hours after sex. Can be inserted only once. Must plan ahead. May slip during intercourse. Some risk of toxic shock	The sponge is moistened with water and inserted into the upper part of the vagina over the cervix.

TABLE 16-2   *Contraceptive Guide (cont.)*

Method	How It Works	Advantages	Disadvantages	How to Use It
SPONGE (*cont.*)	EFFECTIVENESS: 85% AVERAGE COST: $1.75–$3.00 per use.	intercourse. Disposable, one size fits all. Fertility returns immediately upon discontinued use.	syndrome if used incorrectly.	
CONDOM FEMALE	*Reality* female condom prevents sperm from reaching the cervix. It lines the inside of the vagina and covers the cervix, like an inverted male condom. EFFECTIVENESS: 75% AVERAGE COST: $1.50–$3.00 per use.	Protection against sexually transmitted diseases. No prescription needed. Fertility returns immediately upon discontinued use. Allows women to control use. Can be inserted anytime. Safe.	Decreased vaginal sensation. Protrudes outside the vagina which may be distasteful to some couples. One time use.	Place sheath in vagina prior to intercourse.

TABLE 16-2   *Contraceptive Guide (cont.)*

Method	How It Works	Advantages	Disadvantages	How to Use It
CONDOM MALE	Prevents sperm from reaching the cervix. EFFECTIVENESS: 80–90% AVERAGE COST: $0.50–$3.00 per use	No prescription needed. Protects against sexually transmitted diseases. Safe. Fertility returns immediately upon discontinued use.	Can break. Need to plan ahead. Women may be allergic to spermicide or latex. ANIMAL MEMBRANE CONDOMS DO NOT PROTECT AGAINST HIV. Can be used only once. Must be used each time. May interfere with sex.	Condom is placed over an erect penis allowing a pocket at the end to collect sperm.
STERILIZATION MALE	The tube that carries the sperm is cut and then tied or cauterized. This prevents sperm from being ejaculated. No sperm—no pregnancy. Must have	One time decision, doesn't interfere with erection or ejaculation. No known side effects. Doesn't interfere with spontaneity.	Permanent. Surgical procedure required. Some discomfort at the time of the procedure. Only should be chosen if absolutely sure no more children or no children are wanted.	The doctor surgically cuts the vas deferens, or tube that carries the sperm, and then ties it off or cauterizes it.

TABLE 16-2 *Contraceptive Guide (cont.)*

Method	How It Works	Advantages	Disadvantages	How to Use It
STERILIZATION MALE (*cont.*)	two tests before sterility guaranteed. EFFECTIVENESS: 99%+ AVERAGE COST: VARIES			
STERILIZATION FEMALE	Blocking the tube that carries the egg to the uterus either by cutting and tying or by applying cautery, clips or silastic rings. EFFECTIVENESS: 99% AVERAGE COST: VARIES	One time decision. Safe for general health (after procedure). Does not interfere with spontaneity.	Surgical procedure required. Permanent. Less than 1% of women get a rejoining of the tube ends. A very small percentage of women may have increased pain with periods after procedure. Only should be chosen by those that are absolutely sure no children or no	The doctor surgically cuts and ties the tubes through a small incision under the umbilicus after childbirth. A lapsroscope, an instrument inserted through a small abdominal incision, is used to burn the tubes or to place clips or silastic rings over the tubes,

TABLE 16-2 *Contraceptive Guide (cont.)*

Method	How It Works	Advantages	Disadvantages	How to Use It
STERILIZATION FEMALE (*cont.*)			more children are wanted.	thus blocking the tubes.
NATURAL FAMILY PLANNING (RHYTHM)	Refraining from sex during ovulation. EFFECTIVENESS: 75% COST: NONE	No health risks. Approved by the Catholic Church. Can be successful with a highly motivated couple.	Must have good instruction. Must be highly motivated. Day of ovulation unreliable. Must be adhered to on a cycle-to-cycle basis, since a cycle can vary from one month to the next.	Must be aware of how and when ovulation occurs, signs of ovulation, cervical mucus consistency. Most women are fertile a few days before to a few days after ovulation. Ovulation occurs on day 14 in a 28-day cycle; therefore, refrain from sex day 8 to day 18.

Reprinted by permission of Modern Bride (June 1994).

sen and, if there are no contraindications, your doctor should give you a prescription if one is needed.

Any questions you have about your body, sex or emotional problems should be discussed at this visit. If you are planning on having more children, you may wish to discuss how long you should wait before getting pregnant again.

RETURNING TO WORK

You may be very torn about returning to work after the baby is born. Leaving your child can be traumatic for you. Some women have only a six-week maternity leave, while others can take six months or more.

The decision of when to return to work, if you have the flexibility to decide, should be made when it is most comfortable for you, but you should also take your partner's feelings into consideration. Not returning could cause undue financial hardship if you decided to return to work before the baby was born and now change your mind. Your partner may also wish you to stay home as long as possible and you wish to return to work. Discussing the subject before the baby is born will help make the decision easier afterward.

Your baby will miss you when you return to work. Spend time with the baby when you come home. Chores can wait until after the baby is down for a nap or for the night. You have established quiet family time, and you need to continue this practice after you return to work. You also need to have time with your partner. Sometimes you may need to make time.

THE FAMILY

Parenthood is a rewarding and wonderful experience. Enjoy it. You are a family and have begun a journey that will last the rest of your lives.

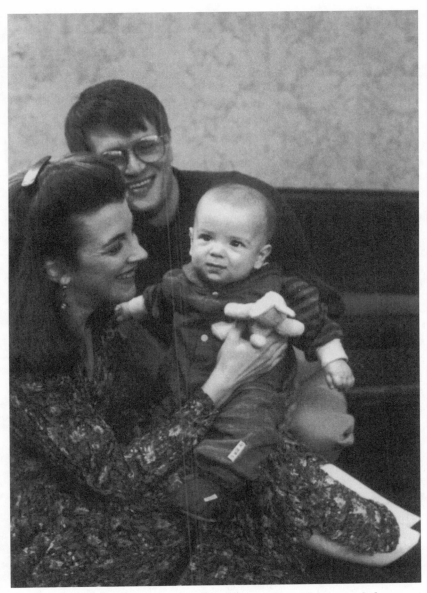

Soon you will not remember what life was like without your baby.

❧ CHAPTER SEVENTEEN

SOME OF US ARE SPECIAL

Special Pregnancies

MULTIPLE BIRTHS

Having more than one baby at a time can come as a shock. It will certainly make your pregnancy more complicated.

TWINS

TYPES

Twins can be identical or fraternal. Identical, or monozygotic, twins are the result of a single fertilized egg dividing into two separate groups of cells early in the initial cell division. Except in rare instances, these twins are the same sex and have exactly the same genetic structure. The rate of identical twins is constant at approximately 4 per 1,000 births.

Fraternal twins are the result of two eggs being fertilized. They can be the same or different sex and have as different a genetic structure as any other two siblings born at different times. The rate of fraternal twins is influenced by maternal age; race; number of previous children, or parity; and where you live. Fraternal twinning increases with maternal age, parity and race. Blacks have more twins than whites; whites have more twins than Asians. The rate of fraternal twins in this country is approximately 8 per 1,000 births.

DIAGNOSIS OF TWINS

Twins are diagnosed by ultrasound. Indications that you may have twins include a uterus larger than it should be, more than one heartbeat and anemia that develops for an unknown reason. If you have taken fertility drugs or had IVF, twins should be suspected until proven otherwise.

If you are carrying twins, you will be more tired and for longer periods than if you were carrying only one baby.

PRENATAL CARE OF TWINS
You should see your doctor more often. Some doctors see twins every two weeks until twenty-eight weeks, then weekly until delivery. Because fundal height is not an accurate measure of fetal growth, ultrasound should be done every four weeks until thirty weeks. After thirty weeks NSTs and biophysical profiles, which assess fetal growth, should be done weekly.

You will need more vitamins and iron during a twin pregnancy. You should take two prenatal vitamins, or a prenatal vitamin plus extra iron. Your calorie intake should also increase an extra 200 to 300 calories. Weight gain in twin pregnancy should be thirty to forty pounds.

Rest at least two hours twice a day after twenty-eight weeks. Work after twenty-eight weeks should be limited to low-stress and minimally strenuous activity.

Twins usually deliver between thirty-six and thirty-seven weeks. Their lungs mature more rapidly than single pregnancies. This may be because of the stress of "crowding" in the uterus. Most twins present head down, or vertex, in labor. If the first twin is head down, your doctor may deliver you vaginally. Both twins are monitored continuously throughout labor. An epidural will usually be given so that rapid c-section can be done if there is a problem in delivery of the second baby. The second twin will be observed on ultrasound as the first baby is delivered. The head of the second baby can then be guided into the pelvis.

COMPLICATIONS OF TWINS
Twins have a higher complication rate than single pregnancies and a higher incidence of preeclampsia and premature labor.

There are also complications that are unique to multiple pregnancies.

"Vanishing Twin." Ultrasound during early pregnancy has revealed a greater frequency of twins than are actually born. There are a number of explanations for this. They include reabsorption of one twin, blighted ovum of one twin and genetic or structural abnormalities that cause growth to stop at an early gestational age. The rate of miscarriage ranges widely, depending on the particular study, from 5 to 40 percent.

Growth Retardation. Twins grow at the same rate as single babies until approximately thirty-two weeks. After thirty-two weeks, the combined weight of the twins is closer to what a single baby would weigh at the same gestational age. This could be the result of crowding or placental insufficiency, which means the placenta cannot keep up with the demands of the babies. Length and the size of each baby's head are close to the size of a single baby.

Discordant Growth. Babies may not be the same size, which can happen in identical twins as a result of what is called twin-twin transfusion. Twin-twin transfusion means that one twin is getting more blood, to the detriment of the other.

Three or More Babies

Because of **IVF** the increased use of fertility drugs, which can cause more than one egg per cycle to be released, we have seen an increase in the number of multiple-fetus pregnancies.

Three or more babies are at even more risk than twins. They deliver much earlier, stop growing at an earlier time during pregnancy and require increased bedrest. Triplets and more are usually delivered by c-section.

Because of the risk of premature delivery and all its attendant complications, a procedure called selective termination has been introduced. A medication is given to a fetus through a needle inserted through the abdomen of the mother, under ultrasound guidance, in the same manner as an amniocentesis is performed. This medication stops the baby's heart. The dead fetus will not cause early delivery or interfere with the continuation of pregnancy. This is a difficult decision to make and should be discussed extensively with your doctor.

MEDICAL PROBLEMS AND PREGNANCY

In the not too distant past, many women who had medical problems could not have children. The risk to mother or baby was considered too great. Now, many women can and do get pregnant. With careful planning, observation and treatment, both mother and baby can do well. You should discuss any medical problems with your doctor.

The following discussion will give you a brief overview of medical problems in pregnancy. Some of these conditions, such as asthma, hypertension, some diabetes and mitral valve prolapse, can be handled by a general obstetrician. Others, such as some diabetes, epilepsy, heart disease, Rh incompatibility and multiple sclerosis, should be handled by an obstetrician with additional training in high-risk obstetrics.

Diabetes

Women with insulin-dependent diabetes used to have a 10 to 30 percent chance of having a stillbirth. With the advent of close maternal and fetal observation, that number has dramatically decreased. Sudden, unexplained stillbirths do still happen, but they are much less common today.

Diabetics are grouped based on the length of time they have had diabetes and whether or not any complications from the disease, such as kidney, vision and vascular problems, have developed. Depending on the severity and class of diabetes, and with optimal control prior to pregnancy, the outcome for your baby can be good. There is an increased rate of fetal structural abnormalities in women who are not well controlled prior to pregnancy. Women who have advanced disease can have poor pregnancy outcomes. Prepregnancy assessment is very important.

Prepregnancy. If your diabetes is controlled by oral medication, you will be placed on insulin injections prior to getting pregnant. The oral medications can cause birth defects and cannot be regulated to control pregnant diabetics. A blood test called a hemoglobin A1C will be done to show the level of control you have on your diabetes.

Treatment in Pregnancy. Your diabetes will be controlled by insulin during pregnancy. Your glucose levels will be kept much lower than when you are not pregnant. This will decrease the risk to your baby.

Prenatal Care. You should be followed extremely closely during pregnancy. You will probably see your doctor on a weekly basis to assess your diabetes. The baby will also be followed closely. NSTs and biophysical profiles will assess the baby beginning at twenty-eight weeks. At thirty-eight weeks, you should have an amniocentesis to determine if the baby's lungs are mature. The lungs of infants of diabetic mothers do not mature as quickly as other babies; therefore, their lungs need to be assessed before delivery.

If the baby's lungs are mature, you will be delivered. If your cervix is ready, you may be induced. You will be given an insulin solution by IV to regulate your glucose level during labor. The baby's glucose is closely related to yours. If yours is increased, the baby's may be decreased.

If you are to have a c-section, you will not need insulin by IV. You should be scheduled early in the morning. Your glucose level will be checked prior to surgery.

The baby will be taken to the intensive care unit to be closely observed.

Complications for Mom. Kidney, vascular or vision problems could become worse during pregnancy. Diabetics are at an increased risk of developing preeclampsia and eclampsia.

Complications for Baby. Infants of diabetic mothers are at an increased risk of developing macrosomia, shoulder dystocia, an inability to regulate glucose, calcium and magnesium, and respiratory distress syndrome if the lungs have not been assessed.

Rh Iso-Immunization (Rh Incompatibility)

An Rh negative mother who has antibodies against Rh positive blood can pass the antibodies to the baby through the placenta. The antibodies can then attack the baby's red blood cells, which carry the Rh antigen.

An Rh iso-immunized pregnancy requires extremely close observation. The baby can have extreme difficulties, including hemolytic anemia, which is anemia caused by the destruction of red blood cells, and intrauterine death.

Prepregnancy. Your antibody titer, the amount of antibody you have, should be assessed as a baseline before you get pregnant. You may have a 60 to 70 percent chance of having an Rh positive baby if your partner is Rh positive. Your obstetric history, including previous pregnancies, is important.

Treatment in Pregnancy/Prenatal Care. Your antibody titer will be assessed frequently by blood tests. Once your titer reaches a critical level, you should have amniocentesis done to assess the severity of the baby's problem. The fluid is tested for bilirubin, a substance made when red blood cells are broken down. If and when the baby is found to be in danger and severely anemic, he may be transfused while still in utero. This is done using ultrasound guidance and transfusing the red blood cells into the baby's abdomen or the umbilical cord. Cordocentesis, transfusing into the umbilical cord, is a relatively new procedure. The baby will be followed closely and, if imminent danger is found, should be delivered. Babies can be delivered as soon as their lungs are mature.

Babies are exchange transfused after birth. This means that their blood is exchanged for fresh, healthy blood. The outcome can be attributed to the improved techniques in transfusing the babies in utero.

Chronic Hypertension

Hypertension, or high blood pressure, is defined as a blood pressure reading of at least 140/90 on several successive determinations. The reason for the hypertension needs to be determined before pregnancy. Most women with hypertension before pregnancy will have essential hypertension, which means the hypertension is not caused by disease.

Chronic hypertension in pregnancy can cause the placental vessels to narrow earlier than in a normal pregnancy. High blood pressure needs to be controlled with medication.

Prepregnancy. You should be assessed for kidney and heart problems caused by the high blood pressure. Laboratory studies should include a baseline urinalysis, electrolytes, serum creatinine, glucose, calcium, baseline uric acid and baseline platelet count.

Treatment in Pregnancy. If you require treatment during pregnancy, your doctor will probably prescribe methyldopa, which is currently the drug of choice. Beta blockers, another type of antihypertensive medication, are also used to control hypertension in pregnancy because, like methyldopa, they do not appear to have an unfavorable effect on the baby.

Prenatal Care. You should be seen more often during your pregnancy. Ultrasounds should be done every four to six weeks beginning at sixteen to twenty weeks. NSTs and biophysical profiles should be done weekly beginning at twenty-eight weeks, with assessment of the placenta. Bedrest may be beneficial from thirty-two to thirty-four weeks until delivery. The baby will be delivered if there is evidence that the placenta is not supplying enough nutrients or oxygen.

Complications for Mom. Mildly hypertensive women are at an increased risk of developing preeclampsia and eclampsia. In addition to these risks, severely hypertensive women can develop kidney failure, stroke, heart failure and abruptio placentae.

Complications for Baby. There is an increased risk of IUGR, prematurity and fetal death. The risk of complications increases with the severity of maternal disease.

Breastfeeding. Diuretics should be avoided, since they suppress lactation. Propranolol, a beta blocker, is not concentrated in breast milk and is considered the drug of choice in treating breastfeeding mothers.

Asthma

Approximately 1 percent of pregnant women have asthma. Pregnancy can make asthma better, worse or have no effect. Each pregnancy is different, and there is no way to predict how your asthma will be affected. You will, however, return to your prepregnancy asthmatic condition by three months postpartum. There appears to be no effect on the baby.

Prepregnancy. You should continue with medications. Most drugs used to treat asthma are considered safe for the baby. Always discuss treatment with your doctor.

Treatment in Pregnancy. Symptomatic asthma should be treated and control should be maintained during pregnancy. Your doctor should treat a severe asthma attack very aggressively.

Prenatal Care. Other than monitoring drug levels to maintain proper levels, your prenatal care should be the same as a pregnant woman without asthma.

Complications for Mom. There appear to be no complications.

Complications for Baby. There appear to be no complications.

Breastfeeding. Discuss the medication you are taking with your doctor to see if it is passed along in breast milk.

Heart Disease

There are various types of heart conditions and each is different in the effect pregnancy may have on it.

Prepregnancy. Pregnant women who are New York Heart Association (NYHA) Class I and II may do well, depending on the specific disease process. Those who are NYHA Class III and IV should not get pregnant, no matter what the disease process.

Treatment in Pregnancy. Treatment should be directed to the specific disease with the risk to the baby taken into account.

Prenatal Care. You should be seen very frequently and observed closely.

Labor and Delivery. An epidural is usually given. Delivery is usually vaginal with forceps assistance to shorten the second stage of labor. The second stage of labor can increase the work the heart is doing, and using forceps to shorten this stage alleviates some of the pressure.

Breastfeeding. This depends on the medication you may be taking. Discuss the possibility of breastfeeding with your doctor.

Mitral Valve Prolapse (MVP)

Women with mitral valve prolapse do well in pregnancy and complications are extremely rare. You need antibiotics in labor and delivery.

Multiple Sclerosis (MS)

Multiple sclerosis is a demyelinating disease, which means that areas of the nerve fibers have lost their protective covering. The cause is unknown and there is no cure. Multiple sclerosis does not affect fertility, and uncomplicated multiple sclerosis has no affect on pregnancy.

Treatment in Pregnancy. If a relapse occurs during pregnancy, a short course of steroids may be given.

Prepregnancy. Medications may be stopped until later in pregnancy.

Prenatal Care. You should be seen more often, and you may need antibiotics frequently since urinary tract infections are increased with some MS patients.

Complications for Mom. There appears to be no increase in complications for mothers with MS.

Complications for Baby. There is an increased chance of the baby developing MS. The risk may be as high as 1 per 100. The risk for the general population is approximately 1 per 1,000.

Breastfeeding. There is no reason not to breastfeed. If you are on medication, discuss the risks with your doctor.

Epilepsy

This is a common neurological disease in which seizures are present. Pregnancy does not change the frequency of seizures in half of all epileptic women. A small percentage of women have fewer seizures, and the balance have more. There is a condition specific to pregnancy called gestational epilepsy. The woman develops generalized seizures usually during the sixth or seventh month. She does not have seizures after the pregnancy, but will develop them again in subsequent pregnancies.

Prepregnancy. Your medication may need to be changed prior to conception since most anticonvulsants cause birth defects. Your doctor should discuss your specific treatment with you.

Treatment in Pregnancy. If treatment is required, your doctor may use phenobarbital, which poses less risk to the baby.

Prenatal Care. You should be seen more frequently. Your anticonvulsant drug levels should be followed closely.

Labor and Delivery. Your doctor should maintain anticonvulsant therapy during labor and delivery.

Breastfeeding. You should be able to breastfeed since very little of the anticonvulsant medication will cross into breast milk; however, this should be discussed with your doctor.

APPENDICES

FOR BABY

Layette
Finding Your Dr. Spock
Questions for Agencies
Agencies
Home Child Care Interview Questions
Questions for Day Care Centers
State Referral Agencies
Babyproofing Your Home

Layette

BATHING BABY
Baby bath/soap
Baby lotion
Baby powder
Baby shampoo
Bathtub with sponge (fitting ring
for later)

CLOTHING
Bonnets/hats
Kimonos
One-piece underwear
Pullover shirts
Side-snap T-shirts
Sleepers
Socks/booties
Sweaters/bunting

GENERAL NEEDS
Activity blanket
Baby book

Baby gym
Bottles, nipples, caps, rings and
bottle sterilizer (even if you
plan to breastfeed)
Breast pump
Brush and comb
Cold pack for trips
Diaper bag
Diaper wipes
High chair
Infant carrier/seat
Nail clippers/scissors
Pacifiers
Playpen
Portable crib
Rattles and toys
Soft-bite spoons/baby
spoons/baby fork
Stroller/carriage
Swing
Teething rings

Unbreakable dishes (cups,
    bowls)
Walker

SAFETY NEEDS
Car seat
Car seat cushions (to hold baby's
    head erect)

LINENS
Bassinet/cradle sheets
Bassinet skirt and liner
Bibs
Changing table cover
Crib sheets (flat and fitted)
Hooded towels
Portable crib sheets
Receiving blankets
Washcloths

MEDICINE CHEST
Activated charcoal (liquid)
Alcohol
Antibiotic ointment (for
    circumcision)
Cotton balls
Cotton swabs
Diaper rash treatment
Infant acetaminophen
Medicine dropper

Petroleum jelly
Rectal thermometer
Syrup of ipecac

NURSERY NEEDS
Bassinet/cradle
Bumper pad for crib
Carryall basket (for diapers,
    wipes, etc.)
Crib
Crib comforter
Crib mattress
Crib mirror
Diapers (cloth/disposable)
Diaper pail
Diaper pins
Diaper stacker
Dresser
Hamper
Humidifier/vaporizer
Mattress protectors (crib and
    bassinet/cradle)
Mobile
Music box
Nightlight/lamp
Nursery monitor
Plastic covers for cloth diapers
Rocking chair
Toy box
Wipes warmer

Finding Your Dr. Spock

The following are suggested questions to use when interviewing a
pediatrician. You should conduct your interview before the baby
is born. Any pediatrician should be happy to meet with you and
answer your questions.

1. Which undergraduate school did you attend?
2. Which medical school did you attend?
3. Where did you do your residency?
4. Why did you choose pediatrics as your specialty?
5. Are you board certified or board eligible?
6. Are you a member of the American Academy of Pediatrics?
7. With which hospitals are you affiliated?
8. What are your office hours?
9. Do you make house calls?
10. Do you have telephone hours? How do you handle phone queries?
11. How are emergencies handled?
12. Solo practitioner: Who is your covering doctor? Does the doctor follow your principles in his or her practice?
13. How are financial matters handled? Which insurance plans do you accept? What are your standard fees?
14. What is your position on breastfeeding? Bottle feeding?
15. What is your position on children's nutrition (e.g., when do you introduce solid foods)? When do you feel vitamins should be given? Fluoride?
16. What is your position on circumcision? What are its pros and cons?
17. When do you think prescription drugs are necessary? Why?
18. What tests do you routinely do after birth? Why?
19. How do you handle jaundice?
20. What are your criteria for early discharge? For rooming in?
21. Breastfeeding: How can you assist us in getting a good start? Can you enforce a "no pacifier/no supplementary bottles" request? Can you facilitate a request for "on demand" feeding?
22. Bottle feeding: Do you have a preference for types of bottle, nipples and formula? Why?
23. Do you recommend specific supplies and equipment? Why?
24. Do you prefer cloth or disposable diapers? Why? Is there a difference in the health of the baby's skin? What are the pros and cons of each?

PEDIATRIC OFFICE OBSERVATION

1. Were you treated courteously, curtly or indifferently on the phone?
2. Upon arrival at the office, were you welcomed cheerfully? Was the receptionist friendly or distant? Were the staff members responsive to and patient with children?
3. Were there age-appropriate toys and books for the children? This will be important as your child grows.
4. Ask parents in the waiting room how long the average wait is. Emergencies do happen, but you should be able to get a good idea. Remember, the personality of the doctor affects the appointment punctuality. A doctor who takes the time to soothe a distraught child is worth the wait.
5. How is the office decorated? Is there child-sized furniture? Is there comfortable furniture for adults? What is the state of the office: tidy with everything in place; dirty/dusty; cluttered with toys and books? Are the children encouraged to play?
6. Does the doctor listen to your questions and what you have to say? Is he or she in a rush to get to the next patient?
7. Although you can expect some guarded answers, especially regarding hospital procedures, is the doctor open and willingly responsive to questions? Remember, the doctor cannot control all hospital policy and employee practices, even though he or she wants to assist you in the best possible manner. Does the doctor solicit questions?
8. Is the doctor fun, compassionate and knowledgeable? Does he or she genuinely appear to like children?

Questions for Agencies

The following are suggested questions to use when interviewing placement agencies for child care help.

1. What is the exact company name?
2. What is your mailing address?
3. How long have you been in business?
4. What geographical area do you cover?
5. What type of caregiver can you provide? Full or part time? Live in or live out?
6. Is there a maximum time frame involved (e.g., one year for an au pair)?
7. How do you screen your prospective child care providers?
8. Are health backgrounds checked?
9. Do you lobby for benefits (paid vacations, medical insurance)?
10. Do you do a background check, including police and credit records?
11. Do you check driver's records?
12. What are the salary ranges you have experienced?
13. Do you offer placement guarantees?
14. Do you place providers with families of children with special needs? What are the requirements for a provider to be placed with special needs children?
15. What is your fee?
16. Do you intervene if specifications are not met on either side?
17. How do you screen your families in search of a provider?
18. Is there anything you would like to add?

Agencies

Below is a list of agencies that specialize in the placement of child care providers.

American Au Pair	Au Pair Registry	Child Care
Boston, MA	Sandy, UT	Placement Service
800/262-8771	800/621-1985	Brookline, MA
		800/338-1836
American Nannies	Boston Nannies, Inc.	
Englewood, NJ	Boston, MA	
201/871-4414	800/648-1351	

Agencies (cont.)

Child Care
Resource and
Referral
Crookston, MN
800/543-7382

Child Care
Solutions
Basking Ridge, NJ
800/752-9653

Children's Choice
Nanny Service
Lester, PA
800/522-4453

Complete Nanny
Limited
Montgomery, NY
800/562-6697

Experiment in Int'l
Living
Au Pair/Homestay
USA
Washington, DC
202/408-5380

Family Exchange
Chestnut Hill, MA
800/545-4592

Harris and
Rothenberg
International
New York, NY
800/323-5594

Heartland Nannies
Registry
North Platte, NE
800/336-9783

Just Nannies
Flanders, NJ
800/752-4811

La Nanny
Fairfax Station, VA
800/526-2669

Maggie's Nanny
Service
Birmingham, AL
800/443-1542

Mother's Helper
Agency
Washington, DC
800/942-2278

Nannies Maid in
Heaven
Merrillville, IN
800/321-6266

Nannies Plus
Livingston, NJ
800/752-0078

Nannies U Trust
Costa Mesa, CA
800/367-2574

Nanny Care
Solutions
800/877-8085

Nanny Factor
Burke, VA
800/232-6269

Nanny Placement
Service
Washington, DC
800/346-2669

North American
Nannies
Ambler, PA
800/343-5316

Notre Maison
Charlotte, NC
800/423-7895

Perfect Nanny
Annapolis, MD
800/882-2698

Playing It Safe
Syosset, NY
800/752-9487

Provider's Choice
Minneapolis, MN
800/356-5983

Whatever Little
Pony Pictures
Riverside, CA
800/367-7747

Home Child Care Interview Questions

The following are suggested questions to use when interviewing a prospective child care provider. Do not be afraid to seek answers to your questions. THIS IS *YOUR* CHILD.

1. Why do you want to take care of children?
2. How long have you been doing this type of work?
3. What is your education level? Have you completed courses on early child development? What was your major course of study?
4. Are you fluent in English? Any other languages?
5. What is your approximate age? (You cannot discriminate on the basis of age.)
6. How many families have you worked for in the past?
7. How many children were in each family and what were their ages?
8. What were your exact duties with each family?
9. Why did you leave those positions?
10. Do you smoke? Drink? Use or ever used illegal drugs?
11. What are your opinions on infant/toddler nutrition?
12. Do you have any special dietary needs? (If your own family has special dietary requirements, these should be explained at this time.) Will this be a problem for you?
13. What is your marital status? Do you have children of your own? If yes, what are their ages? Who cares for them while you are with my child? Would there ever be a time when your child/children came to work with you? (This is for live-out positions.)
14. What is your religion? (This is the time to explain your own family's religious beliefs and ascertain whether there would be a problem for the candidate.)
15. As my child gets older, what methods of behavior encouragement/discouragement would you use? What do you believe are good disciplinary tactics?

16. Do you feel you are reliable?
17. Are you punctual?
18. What would you do if my child were injured in your care?
19. Do you know infant CPR? If yes, when does your certificate expire? If no, would you learn?
20. What do you consider an emergency?
21. Would you sign an employment contract? For how long? If no, why?
22. Will you authorize a police background check and a credit check? If no, why?
23. Will you authorize a driver's record investigation? If no, why?
24. What is your Social Security number?
25. What is your current address? Telephone number?
26. May we contact your previous employers? (Get names and telephone numbers.) If no, why?
27. What salary do you expect? Benefits?
28. What are your hobbies? Interests?

Questions for Day Care Centers

The following are suggested questions and observations for you to consider when searching for a day care center. Even though most of these items appear to be geared to older children, remember that your newborn will grow. Also, by using these items as a checklist, you will get an overall sense of how the facility is run.

Are you a licensed facility?

When was your license issued?

Is the license current? (Ask for a copy of the license to take home with you.)

Do you have insurance coverage?

Who is the carrier?

What is the subscriber listed as (name of center or individual)?

What type of policy is it?

What are its coverage points (damages, medical, liability, etc.)?

How long have you been caring for children?

How many children are in the program? Full time? Part time?

What is the total square footage of the facility?

What is the square footage used by children?

Does the provider have children? How many? Ages?

Are they at the home/facility during the day?

What training does each provider have?

Where did the provider receive her or his education and degree?

What first aid training do the providers have? (Obtain copies of first aid training certificates.)

Where are first aid supplies kept?

With which agencies are you affiliated?

Is there backup available if any provider is ill or on vacation?

What ages do you care for?

What hours of care are provided?

Who operates the center? Administrators? Child care providers?

How many providers are at the facility at any given time?

What is the maximum size of the group?

What type of program is offered—developmental, custodial, mini-nursery?

How long has each caregiver been with the program?

What are the qualifications of the caregivers?

What are the ages of the caregivers?

What is your maximum staff/child ratio?

What is your illness policy?

Are meals or snacks provided?

What is a typical weekly menu?

What emergency room is used in the event of an emergency?

What is your philosophy on parental involvement?

What are your policies on toilet training? Bottles? Pacifiers?

What is the educational philosophy of the center?

Do the providers participate in continuing education programs to sharpen their skills?

What is the minimum number of adults on duty at any point on any given day?

What days is the center closed?

What are the evacuation plans in case of a fire?

Are there fire drills?

Is there more than one exit available?

Are health records maintained?

Is there an open visitation policy?

What activities are offered?

What is the core curriculum?

What types of records are maintained on the children, other than financial?

What discipline methods are used? (Ask for a list of references.)

Are you a member of the Better Business Bureau or the local Chamber of Commerce?

Has your license ever been under investigation?

In the past five years, have there been any legal claims filed against your center? If yes, why? Outcome?

TAKE NOTE OF THE FOLLOWING

General facility: Is it clean and in good repair?

Is there good light and ventilation?

Are there safety guards on the windows?

Are there smoke detectors? Fire extinguishers? Location of each?

Is there more than one way out in case of a fire?

Are there covers on electrical outlets?

Are there covers on radiators?

Are there safety gates on stairs?

Are there clean, friendly pets (if applicable)?

Is there a defined outside play area?

Is the area free of hazards? Equipment in good condition? Area fenced?

Is there grass, rubber or sand on the play surface?

Is the layout structured for easy view of all the children from all vantage points?

Are the fence gates latched? In good working order?

Is there a pool, stream, pond on the property? Are these accessible to the children?

Are active play area and quiet play area separated inside the facility?

Is there a variety of age-appropriate toys?

Is there a television? How is it utilized (to keep children quiet or for educational purposes)?

OBSERVATIONS

PLAY EQUIPMENT: Is it dirty, in disrepair, clean, well used? Does it seem safe? Is outdoor equipment well anchored and free of debris, rusting bolts, holes? Are bikes, scooters and other items in good repair? Are toys in good repair, in proper working order, safety tested?

MEAL/SNACK FACILITIES: Is the space adequate to accommodate all the children? Are the utensils, dishes, tables and chairs geared to children, or do the children eat from paper plates or glass dishes? Is the kitchen and cooking area clean and well maintained?

BATHROOMS: Are facilities available for children who are able to use them without assistance (smaller toilets or step-up systems)? Is there more than one potty chair, or do all children being trained use the same potty? Are the potty chair and toilet kept clean? Do children and providers wash their hands after toilet activities?

CHANGING AREAS: Are there safety straps on the changing table? Are diaper pails kept closed? Are items within reach of provider so child is not left unattended? Do providers wash their hands after changing each diaper?

REST AREAS: Are there cribs or beds for children who take naps? Is there a separate crib for each infant, or do infants share cribs? Are the linens clean? Are cribs in good repair? Are beds suitable for children? If there are no beds, where do children who are no longer in cribs take their naps? If there are no cribs, where do infants take there naps? Are playpens used for play or naps?

*Day Care Referral Services**

Capable Care
Washington, DC
800/262-6697

Kids Unlimited Service
Charlton, MA
800/422-6738

*See also State Referral Agencies listing

State Referral Agencies

If your state is not listed, check the Yellow Pages under GOVERNMENT (both state and local).

Alabama Association for Child
  Care Resource and Referral
  Agencies
309 N. 23rd St.
Birmingham, AL 35203
205/252-1991

Alaska Child Care Resource
  and Referral Alliance
P.O. Box 10339
Anchorage, AK 99510
907/279-5024

California Child Care Resource
and Referral Network
809 Lincoln Way
San Francisco, CA 94122
415/661-1714

Colorado Child Care Resource
and Referral Network
5675 S. Academy Blvd.
Colorado Springs, CO 80906
715/540-7252

Florida Child Care Resource
and Referral Network
1282 Paul Russel Rd.
Tallahassee, FL 32301
904/656-2272

Illinois Child Care Resource
and Referral System
100 W. Randolph
Suite 16-206
Chicago, IL 60601
312/814-5524

Indiana Association for Child
Care Resource and Referral
4460 Guion Rd.
Indianapolis, IN 46254
317/299-2750

Iowa Commission on Children,
Youth and Families
Department of Human
Rights
Lucas Building
Des Moines, IA 50319
515/281-3974

Maine Association of Child
Care Resource and
Referral Agencies
P.O. Box 280-WHCA
Millbridge, ME 04658
207/546-7544

Maryland Child Care Resource
Network
608 Water Street
Baltimore, MD 21202
301/752-7588

Massachusetts Office for
Children
10 West St.
Fifth Floor
Boston, MA 02111
617/727-8900

Michigan Community
Coordinated Child Care
Association
2875 Northwind Dr.
#200
East Lansing, MI 48823
517/351-4171

Minnesota Child Care Resource
and Referral Network
2116 Campus Dr. SE
Rochester, MN 55904
507/287-2497

New Hampshire Association of
Child Care Resource and
Referral Agencies
99 Hanover St.
P.O. Box 448
Manchester, NH 03105
317/299-2750

New Jersey Statewide
Clearinghouse
Division of Youth and Family
Services
50 E. State St.
CN 717
Trenton, NJ 08625
609/292-8408

New York State Child Care
Coordinating Council
237 Bradford St.
Albany, NY 12206
518/463-6697

North Carolina Child Care
Resource and Referral
Network
700 Kenilworth Ave.
Charlotte, NC 28204
704/376-6697

Ohio Child Care Resource and
Referral Association
92 Jefferson Ave.
Columbus, OH 43215
614/224-0222

Oregon Child Care Resource
and Referral Network
325 Thirteenth St.
Suite 206
Salem, OR 97301
503/585-6232

South Carolina Child Care
Resource and Referral
Network
2129 Santee Ave.
Columbia, SC 29205
803/254-9263

Texas Association of Child Care
Resource and Referral
Agencies
4029 Capital of Texas Hwy. S.
Suite 102
Austin, TX 78704
512/440-8555

Vermont Association of Child
Care Resource and Referral
Agencies
Vermont College
Montpelier, VT 05602
802/828-8675

Virginia Child Care Resource
and Referral Network
3701 Pender Dr.
Fairfax, VA 22030

Washington State Child Care
Resource and Referral
Network
P.O. Box 1241
Tacoma, WA 98401
206/383-1735

Wisconsin Child Care
Improvement Project
315 West 5th
P.O. Box 369
Hayward, WI 54843
715/634-3905

Babyproofing Your Home

The following is a list of suggestions for babyproofing your home. For further assistance, contact the local affiliate of Baby Proofers International for a home inspection.

To fireproof linens and clothing, combine nine ounces of borax, four ounces of boric acid solution and one gallon of warm water. Soak clean clothes and linens in the solution until completely wet. Wring, then dry as usual.

Put cleaning supplies and chemicals out of reach.

Throw away dry cleaning bags.

Relock high chair tray when you take your child out of the seat.

Popcorn, nuts, raisins and peanut butter on a spoon can cause choking. Don't feed them to a young child.

Keep your house or apartment free of loose rugs.

Always keep outside doors locked.

Make sure all equipment has the Juvenile Products Manufacturers Association's safety certification seal.

Check with your local police department regarding fingerprinting your child as a safety precaution.

Watch your child in unfamiliar surroundings.

Do not use lawn mowers or power tools around your child.

Teach your child to pick up any toys to prevent accidents.

NEVER leave an infant or young child alone in the tub.

Don't tie a pacifier around your child's neck.

Put "Tot Finder" decals on your child's bedroom window and the outside door of your home or apartment.

Keep trash out of reach.

Keep small electrical appliances in bathrooms unplugged when not in use.

Don't use curling irons, blow dryers or other bathroom appliances around your child.

Put plastic caps over electrical outlets.

Put electrical cords from lamps and appliance out of reach.

Keep toothpicks, needles, pins, knives, scissors and other sharp objects out of reach.

Put window guards on all windows and close stairways with gates that are securely fastened to the wall.

Secure cupboards with childproof locks.

Put covers on all doorknobs.

Check all freestanding shelves for stability.

Keep appliances securely locked.

Put locks on toilets.

Block tape slot on VCR so your child can't stick fingers or objects into it.

Paste down rubber tips of doorstops.

Put padded bumpers on sharp corners of tables and cabinets.

Put a gate across doorways you don't want your child to cross.

Block the stairs with gates or netting devices.

Keep space heaters out of reach.

Keep pot handles turned to the back of the stove.

Boil and fry foods on the back burners.

Sweep up broken glass with a wet paper towel.

Keep liquor out of reach. Alcohol can be extremely toxic to a young child.

Reduce the temperature on the hot water heater.

Put faucet protectors over tub faucet, even if your baby is still in an infant bath or bath ring.

Use only paper or plastic cups in the bathroom.

Keep razors, medicines and vitamins out of reach.

Do not let your child play in the bathroom.

Fix bathroom doors so that only an adult can lock them.

Use proper infant carriers and car seats in automobiles.

Use helmets and proper child carriers when biking.

Use place mats instead of tablecloths.

Put a nonslip pad or decals on the bottom of your tub.

Keep a first aid kit on hand.

Keep matches and lighters out of reach.

Equip your home with fire extinguishers and smoke detectors.

Store flammable liquids in tightly capped containers clearly marked. Keep away from heating unit.

Keep your child out of the kitchen when you're cooking.

Don't heat bottles in a microwave.

Put lighted candles where they can't be knocked down.

Keep flashlights instead of candles for power outages.

Avoid overloading electrical outlets.

Replace frayed cords.

Turn off all lights before going to bed.

Keep appliances in good working order.

NEVER put water on an electrical fire.

Cover all radiators.

SAFETY EQUIPMENT

Doorstops

Doorknob covers

Drawer stops

Outlet covers

Safety gate

Stair rail netting for staircase spindles

Stove guard

Toilet locks

RECOMMENDED READING

Safe Kids: A Complete Child-Safety Handbook and Resource Guide for Parents by Vivian Kramer Fancher, 1991

FOR DAD

Support Groups
Books
Videos

For Dad

The following may be helpful resources.

SUPPORT GROUPS
Fatherhood Project
c/o Families and Work Institutes
330 Seventh Ave.
Fourteenth Floor
New York, NY 10001
212/268-4846

Father's Resource Center
423 Oak Grove St.
Suite 105
Minneapolis, MN 55403
612/874-1509

BOOKS
Between Father and Child by Dr. Ronald Levant and John Kelly, 1989
Birth of a Father by Dr. Martin Greenberg, 1985
Daddy's Home by Greg Johnson and Mike Yorkey, 1992
The Expectant Father by Connie Marshall, R.N., 1992
The Father Book: An Instruction Manuel by Drs. Frank Minirth, Bryan
    Newman, Paul Warren, 1992
The Father's Almanac by S. Adams Sullivan, 1992
How to Be a Pregnant Father by Peter Mayle and Arthur Robins, 1993

The Thirteen Months of Pregnancy: A Guide for the Pregnant Father by Bill
   M. Atalla, 1992
When Men Are Pregnant: Needs and Concerns of Expectant Fathers by
   Jerrold Lee Shapiro, Ph.D., 1987

VIDEOS
The Expectant Father Video
For information, contact:
The Family Room
P.O. Box 4481
Troy, MI 48099
800/745-1145

FOR MOM

Support Groups
Magazines
Maternity Wear
Your Suitcase
Books/Videos/Music Boxes

Support Groups

The following is a list of resources you may find helpful before, during and after your pregnancy.

AT-HOME MOMS
FEMALE (Formerly Employed
   Mother at the Leading Edge)
P.O. Box 31
Elmhurst, IL 60126
708/941-3553

Mothers at Home
P.O. Box 2208
Merrifield, VA 22116
703/352-2292

Mothers Matter
171 Wood St.
Rutherford, NJ 07070
201/933-8191

National Association of Mothers
   Centers
800/645-3828

BEDREST PREGNANCIES
Confinement Line
c/o The Childbirth Education
   Association
P.O. Box 1609
Springfield, VA 22151
703/941-7183

CESAREAN SECTION
Cesarean Prevention
   Movement
P.O. Box 152
Syracuse, NY 13210
315/424-1942

C/SEC (Cesarean/Support,
   Education and Concern)
22 Forest Rd.
Framingham, MA 01701

FEEDING BABY
Formula
P.O. Box 39051
Washington, DC 20016
703/527-7171

Human Lactation Center
666 Sturges Hwy.
Westport, CT 06880
203/259-5995

Infant Formula
5775 Peachtree Dunwoody Rd.
Suite 500-D
Atlanta, GA 30342
404/252-3663

International Baby Food
  Action Network
c/o Action
3255 Hennepin Ave. S.
Suite 220
Minneapolis, MN 55408
612/823-1571

International Lactation
  Consultant Association
P.O. Box 4031
University of Virginia Station
Charlottesville, VA 22903
404/879-1137

LaLeche League
9616 Minneapolis Ave.
Franklin Park, IL 60131
800/LALECHE

GENERAL
Child Help USA
800/422-4453

National Association of
  Postpartum Care Services
  (Doulas)
4414 Buxton Court
Indianapolis, IN 46254
317/293-7763

Parents Anonymous
800/421-0353

MEDITATION
The International Society
  of Love
P.O. Box 1804
Makawao, HI 96768
808/572-2368

MULTIPLES
International Twins Association
c/o Marilyn Holms
511 Gilpin St.
Denver, CO 80209

National Organization of
  Mothers of Twins Club
12404 Princess Jeanne, N.E.
Albuquerque, NM 87112
505/275-0955

Triplet Connection
P.O. Box 99571
Stockton, CA 95209
209/474-0885

Twins Foundation
P.O. Box 6043
Providence, RI 02940
401/274-TWIN

POSTPARTUM
Depression after Delivery
P.O. Box 1285
Morrisville, PA 19067
215/295-3994

Postpartum Support
  International
927 Kellogg Ave.
Santa Barbara, CA 93111
805/967-7636

SINGLE MOMS
Parents without Partners
8807 Colesville Rd.
Silver Spring, MD 20910
301/588-9354

Single Mothers by Choice
P.O. Box 1642
Gracie Square Station
New York, NY 10028
212/988-0993

Single Parent Resource
  Center
1165 Broadway
Room 504
New York, NY 10001
212/213-0047

WORKING MOMS
Catalyst
250 Park Avenue S.
New York, NY 10003
212/777-8900

Magazines

American Baby
P.O. Box 53093
Boulder, CO 80322-3093
800/525-0643

Baby Talk
636 Avenue of the Americas
New York, NY 10011
212/989-8187

Child
P.O. Box 3173
Harlan, IA 51593-2364
800/777-0222

Consumer Reports
256 Washington St.
Mount Vernon, NY 10553-1099
914/667-9400

Exceptional Parent Magazine
  (for parents of special
  needs children)
Department EP
P.O. Box 3000
Denville, NJ 07834-9199
201/730-5800

Expecting
685 Third Ave.
29th Floor
New York, NY 10017-4024
212/878-8700

Growing Child
22 N. Second St.
P.O. Box 620
Lafayette, IN 47902-0620
317/423-2624

Lamaze Parents Magazine
1840 Wilson Blvd.
Suite 204
Arlington, VA 22201-3000

Mothering
P.O. Box 532
Mount Morris, IL 61054
800/545-9364

Mothers Today
18 E. 41st St.
New York, NY 10017-6237
212/481-9030

Parenting
P.O. Box 53434
Boulder, CO 80321-2424
800/727-3682

Parents
P.O. Box 3055
Harlan, IA 51593-2364
800/727-3682

Twins Magazine
P.O. Box 12045
Overland Park, KS 66212
800/821-5533

Working Mother
P.O. Box 53841
Boulder, CO 80321-3841
303/447-9330

Working Parents
18 E. 41st St.
New York, NY 10017-6222
212/481-9030

Working Woman
342 Madison Ave.
New York, NY 10173-0008
212/309-9800

Maternity Wear

The following is a list of national chain maternity stores that offer basic as well as alternative maternity wear. Call for the store in your area.

Dansu Creations
Bensalem, PA
800/258-0082

Dill Pickle Maternity
Spokane, WA
800/321-3455

Maternity Wearhouse
Philadelphia, PA
800/872-6667

MOTHERHOOD
Santa Monica, CA
800/277-1903

Mother's Work
Philadelphia, PA
215/625-9259

Pea in a Pod
Irving, TX
800/594-6888

Page Boy Maternity
Dallas, TX
800/225-3103

Reborn Maternity
New York, NY
212/737-8817

Recreations Maternity
Columbus, OH
800/621-2547

Your Suitcase

The following items should be packed in your hospital suitcase or bag. You should have this ready at the end of your seventh month. Pack enough for a three-day stay, even if you are planning on a twenty-four-hour discharge. Remember, the baby may have its own agenda.

FOR MOM

CLOTHES
Nightgowns
Nursing bras
Panties
Robe
Slippers
An outfit to wear home

TOILETRIES
Comb
Deodorant
Hairbrush
Hair dryer
Makeup
Shampoo
Soap (unscented)

Toothbrush
Toothpaste

MISCELLANEOUS
Bottled mineral water
Camera and extra film
Saltines
Suckers/lollipops
"To call" telephone list
Tea bags (herbal)
Birthing plan
Hospital papers
Insurance documentation
A novel or magazine to read
A bottle of champagne or
   sparkling cider for celebrating
   and glasses

FOR DAD
Snacks

FOR BABY
Baby book
Clothes for the trip home
Diapers

Books/Videos/Music Boxes

These resources may be helpful as you continue to learn and prepare for the new baby.

BOOKS

Breastfeeding Today by Candace Woessner, Judith Lauwers and Barbara Bernard, 1991

Child Care: A Parent's Guide by Sonja Flating, 1991

A Child Is Born by Leonart Nilsson, 1990

Creative Visualizations by Shakti Gawain

Curse of the Mommy by Cathy Crimmins, 1993

Dictionary of First Names by Alfred J. Kolatch, 1990

Empty Arms: Coping with Miscarriage, Stillbirth and Infant Death by Sherokee Ilse, 1989

Essential Exercises for the Childbearing Years, 3rd ed. by Elizabeth Noble, 1988

From Aaron to Zoe: 15,000 Great Baby Names by Daniel Avram Richman, 1993

How to Hire a Nanny by Elaine S. Pelletier, 1994

Lamaze Is for Chickens: A Guide to Prepared Childbirth by Mimi Green and Maxine Naab, 1985

Books (*cont.*)

Miracle Baby by Mark Perloe, M.D., and Linda Gail Christie, 1986

Mother Massage by Elaine Stillerman, L.M.T., 1992

Mother Murphy's Law and Other Perils of Parenthood by Bruce Lansky, 1986

Painless Childbirth by Dr. Fernand Lamaze, 1984

Pregnant Feelings: Developing Trust in Birth by R. Baldwin and T. Richardson

Pregnant Woman's Comfort Guide by Sherry L. M. Jimenez, R.N., 1992

Suzy Prudden's Pregnancy and Back to Shape Exercise Program by Suzy Prudden and Jeffrey Sussman, 1980

The Best Baby Name Book in the Whole World by Bruce Lansky

The Guide to Baby Products, 3rd rev. ed. by Sandy Jones, 1991

The Womanly Art of Breastfeeding, 5th rev. ed. by LaLeche League International, 1991

The Working Woman's Lamaze Handbook by Robin Sweet and Patty Bryan, 1992

The Worst Baby Name Book by Bob Glickman, 1990

Yoga for Pregnancy by Sandra Jordan, 1987

Your Premature Baby by Frank P. Mangiello, M.D., and Theresa Fay, 1991

VIDEOS

Jane Fonda's *Workout for Pregnancy, Birth and Recovery*

Tracy Schmidt's *Every Mom's Prenatal Exercise Video*

Kathy Smith's *Pregnancy Workout*

MUSIC BOXES

Rita Ford Music Boxes, Inc.
19 E. 65th St.
New York, NY 10021
212/535-6717

The San Francisco Music Box Company
(This is a national chain; check local listings)

FOR BIG BROTHER/SISTER

Books for Big Brother/Sister
Books about Siblings

The following resources may be helpful for preparing siblings for the new baby. Also check out sibling classes at the location you have chosen to have the baby.

Books for Big Brother/Sister

Arthur's Baby by Marc Brown
Babies by Dorothy Hinshaw Patent, 1988
A Baby for Max by Kathryn Lasky and Maxwell Knight, 1984
Baby's Book of Babies by Kathy Henderson and Anthea Sieveking, 1989
Before You Were Born by Margaret Sheffield and Sheila Bewley, 1984
Being Born by Sheila Kitzinger and Lennart Nilsson, 1986
Born Two-Gether by Jan Brennan
Brothers and Sisters by Maxine B. Rosenberg, 1991
Getting Ready for the New Baby by Harriett Ziefert and Laura Rodar
Hard to Be Six by Arnold Adoff
How You Were Born by Joanna Cole, 1984
It's a Baby by George Ancona, 1985
Let Me Tell You about My Baby by Roslyn Banish, 1988
Love You Forever by Robert Munsch, 1986
The New Baby by Fred Rogers and Jim Jenkins, 1974
Nobody Asked Me If I Wanted a Baby Sister by Martha Alexander
Peter's Chair by Ezra Jack Keats
The Stork Didn't Bring Me by Marie Francine Herbert
We Are Having a Baby by Viki Holland
We Got This New Baby at Our House by Janet Sinberg and Nancy Gray, 1980

Books about Siblings

He Hit Me First by Louise Bates Ames, Ph.D., 1985
Siblings without Rivalry by Adele Faber and Elaine Mazlish, 1987
Sibling Rivalry by Seymour V. Reit, 1985

❧ APPENDIX 5

MATERNITY LEAVE

The following organizations are helpful resources for information on maternity leave and your rights.

National Employment
   Opportunity Commission
2401 East St. N.W.
Room 500
Washington, DC
202/634-6700

National Organization for
   Women
100 Sixteenth St., N.W.
Suite 700
Washington, DC 20036
202/331-0066

9 to 5, the National Association
   of Working Women
614 Superior Avenue, N.W.
Room 852
Cleveland, OH 44113
800/245-9865

Women's Legal Defense Fund
2000 P St., N.W.
Washington, DC 20036
202/887-0364

Women's Rights Projects
American Civil Liberties Union
132 W. 43rd St.
New York, NY 10036
212/944-9800

NATIONAL ORGANIZATIONS

The following list of national organizations can be used as a resource guide.

BEREAVEMENT/GRIEF
Grief Education Institute
Suite 132
Denver, CO 80222
302/758-6048

Local chapters of
  Compassionate Friends
  Jewish Family Services
  Catholic Charities Family
    Services

BIRTHING CENTERS
CHOICE (Center for Humane
  Options in Childbirth
  Experience)
54426 Madison St.
Hilliard, OH 43026
617/771-0863

Maternity Center Association
48 E. Ninety-second St.
New York, NY 10128
212/369-7300

(International Association of
  Parents and Professionals for
  Safe Alternatives in
  Childbirth)
Route 1
Box 646
Marble Hill, MO 63764
314/238-2010

National Association of
  Childbearing Centers
3123 Gottschall Rd.
Perkiomenville, PA 18075

CHILDBIRTH EDUCATION
American Academy of Husband
  Coached Childbirth (Bradley
  method)
P.O. Box 5224
Sherman Oaks, CA 86336
800/423-2397
818/788-6662

American Society of Childbirth
  Educators
P.O. Box 1630
Sedona, AZ 86336
602/284-9897

ASPO (Lamaze method)
1101 Connecticut Ave., N.W.
Suite 700
Washington, DC 20036
800/368-4404
202/857-1128

Childbirth Education
  Foundation
P.O. Box 5
Richboro, PA 18954
215/357-2792

Childbirth without Pain
  Education Association
  (Lamaze method)
20134 Snowden
Detroit, MI 48235
313/341-3816

International Childbirth
  Education Association
P.O. Box 20048
Minneapolis, MN 55420
612/854-8660

Midwest Parentcraft Center
  (Gamper method)
3921 N. Lincoln
Chicago, IL 60613
312/281-6638

Read Natural Childbirth
  Foundation
P.O. Box 956
San Rafael, CA 94915
415/456-8462

CHILD SAFETY
Child Find of America
P.O. Box 277
New Paltz, NY 12561
914/255-1848

Consumer Product Safety
  Commission
5401 Westbard Ave.
Bethesda, MD 20207
301/492-6800

Environmental Protection
  Agency
401 M. St., S.W.
Washington, DC 20460
202/382-2090

Juvenile Products Manufacturers
  Association
Two Greentree Centre
Suite 225
Marlton, NJ 08053
609/985-2878

National Highway Traffice Safety
  Administration (car seat info)
800/424-9393
202/366-0123

National Institute for
Occupational Safety and
Health
4676 Columbia Pkwy.
Cincinnati, OH 45226
800/356-4674

National Safety Council
444 Michigan Ave.
Chicago, IL 60611-3991
312/527-4800

National Sudden Infant Death
Syndrome
10500 Little Paterxent Pkwy.
Suite 420
Columbia, MD 21044
800/221-7437
301/459-3388

National Resources Defense
Council (Mothers and Others
for a Livable Planet)
40 W. Twentieth St.
New York, NY 10011
212/727-2700

Occupational Safety and Health
Administration
200 Constitution Ave., N.W.
Washington, DC 20210
202/523-8148

Toy Manufacturers of America,
Inc.
200 Fifth Ave.
New York, NY 10010
212/675-1141

FAMILY PHYSICIANS
American Academy of Family
Physicians
8880 Ward Pkwy.
Kansas City, MO 64114
816/333-9700

American Board of Family
Practice
2228 Young Dr.
Lexington, KY 40505
606/269-5626

American College of Medicine
233 E. Erie St.
Suite 710
Chicago, IL 60611
312/951-1400

GENERAL
Al-Anon
P.O. Box 862
Midtown Station
New York, NY 10018
212/302-7240

Alcoholics Anonymous
P.O. Box 459
Grand Central Station
New York, NY 10163
212/683-3900

American Association for
Marriage and Family Therapy
1717 K St., N.W.
Suite 407
Washington, DC 20006
202/452-0109

American Board of Medical
  Genetics
9650 Rockville Pike
Bethesda, MD 20814
301/571-1825

American Diabetes Association
1660 Duke St.
Alexandria, VA 22314
800/232-3472

American Foundation for
  Maternal and Child Health
439 E. Fifty-first St.
New York, NY 10022
212/759-5510

American Medical Association
515 N. State St.
Chicago, IL 60640

Drug-Anon
443 W. Fiftieth St.
New York, NY
212/484-9095

Emotions Anonymous
P.O. Box 4245
St. Paul, MN 55104
612/647-9712

Family Service America
11700 W. Lake Park Dr.
Milwaukee, WI 53224-3099
414/359-2111

Healthy Mothers, Healthy
  Babies
409 Twelfth St., S.W.
Room 309
Washington, DC 20024
202/863-2458

International Association for
  Medical Assistance to Travelers
417 Center St.
Lewiston, NY 14092
716/754-4883

The International Nanny
  Association
P.O. Box 26522
Austin, TX 78755-0522
512/454-6462

National Academy of Nannies,
  Inc.
3300 E. First Ave.
Suite 520
Denver, CO 80206
303/333-NANI

National Association for Family
  Daycare
815 Fifteenth St.
Suite 928
Washington, DC 20005
202/347-3356

National Association for Sickle
  Cell Disease
4221 Wilshire Blvd.
Suite 360
Los Angeles, CA 90010
800/421-8453

National Association of Genetic
  Counsellors
233 Canterbury Dr.
Wallingford, PA 19086
215/872-7608

National Clearinghouse for
  Maternal and Child Health
Thirty-eighth and R Streets, N.W.
Washington, DC 20057
202/625-8410

National Genetics Foundation
P.O. Box 1374
New York, NY 10101

National Health Information
  Center
P.O. Box 1133
Washington, DC 20013
800/336-4797
301/565-4167

National Institute of Child
  Health and Human
  Development
NIH Building 31
Room 2A32
Rockville, MD 20892
301/496-5133

National Mental Health
  Association
1021 Prince St.
Alexandria, VA 22314
703/684-7722

National Multiple Sclerosis
  Society
205 E. Forty-second St.
New York, NY 10017-5706
212/986-3240

National Organization of
  Circumcision Information
  Resource Center
P.O. Box 2512
San Anselmo, CA 94960
415/488-9883

Newborn Rights Society
P.O. Box 48
St. Peters, PA 19470
215/353-6061

Non-Circumcision Education
  Foundation
P.O. Box 5
Richmond, PA 18954
215/357-2792

Non-Circumcision Information
  Center
P.O. Box 31
Waverly, MA 02179
617/489-4530

Peaceful Beginnings
13020 Homestead Court
Anchorage, AK 99516
907/345-4813

Remain Intact Organization
RR 2 Box 86
Larchwood, IA 51241
172/477-2256

HOME BIRTH
American College of Home
  Obstetrics
P.O. Box 508
Oak Park, IL 60303
708/383-1461

Association for Childbirth at
  Home, International
P.O. Box 430
Glendale, CA 91209
213/667-0839
213/663-4996

Informed Homebirth/Informed
  Parenting
P.O. Box 3675
Ann Arbor, MI 48106
313/662-6857

HOSPITALS
American Hospital Association
840 N. Lake Shore Dr.
Chicago, IL 60611
312/280-6000

INFERTILITY
American Fertility Society
1209 Montgomery Hwy.
Birmingham, AL 35216
205/978-5000

RESOLVE—Infertility Education
8100 Mountain Rd. N.E.
Albuquerque, NM 87110
505/266-1170

MASSAGE
American Massage Therapy
  Association
820 Davis St.
Suite 100
Evanston, IL 60201
708/864-0123

MIDWIVES
American College of Nurse-
  Midwives
1552 K St., N.W.
Suite 1000
Washington, DC 20005
202/289-0171

Midwives Alliance of North
  America
P.O. Box 1121
Bristol, VA 24203-1121
615/764-5561

OBSTETRICIANS
American Board of Obstetrics
  and Gynecology
4225 Roosevelt Way N.E.
Suite 305
Seattle, WA 98105
206/547-4884

American College of
  Obstetricians and
  Gynecologists
409 Twelfth St., S.W.
Washington, DC 20023-2188
202/638-5577

American Gynecological and
  Obstetrical Society
50 N. Medical Dr.
University of Utah
Salt Lake City, UT 84132
801/581-5501

OSTEOPATHS
American College of General
  Practitioners in Osteopathic
  Medicine and Surgery
330 E. Algonquin Rd.
Arlington Heights, IL 60005
708/228-6090

American Osteopathic
  Association
142 E. Ontario St.
Chicago, IL 60611
312/280-5800

PEDIATRICIANS
American Academy of Pediatrics
41 Northwest Point Blvd.
Box 927
Elk Grove Village, IL 60009
312/228-5005

American Board of Pediatrics
111 Silver Cedar Court
Chapel Hill, NC 27514
919/929-0461

American Pediatric Society
Johns Hopkins Hospital
400 N. Wolfe St.
CMSC2-124
Baltimore, MD 21205
301/955-2727

❧ APPENDIX 7

SPECIAL NEEDS CHILDREN

The following is a list of national organizations and clearinghouses that provide information on resources available for special needs children and their parents. Contact them to learn about resources in your area.

American Council of Rural
   Special Education
Department of Special
   Education
University of Utah
Milton Bennison Hall
Salt Lake City, UT 84112
801/581-8442

American Foundation
   for the Blind
15 W. Sixteenth St.
New York, NY 10011
800/232-5463
212/620-2000
212/620-2158 (TDD)

American Occupational
   Therapy Association
P.O. Box 1725
1383 Piccard Dr.
Rockville, MD 20849-1725
301/948-9626

American Physical Therapy
   Association
1111 N. Fairfax St.
Alexandria, VA 22314
703/684-2782

American Speech-Language-
   Hearing Association
10801 Rockville Pike
Rockville, MD 20852
800/638-8255
301/897-5700

Association for Children with
   Retarded Mental Development
162 Fifth Ave.
Eleventh Floor
New York, NY 10010
212/741-0100

Association for Persons with
   Severe Handicaps
11201 Greenwood Ave. N.
Seattle, WA 98133
206/361-8870
206/361-0113 (TDD)

Association for the Advancement
of Rehabilitation Technology
1101 Connecticut Ave., N.W.
Suite 700
Washington, DC 20036
202/857-1199

Association for the Care of
Children's Health
7910 Woodmont Ave.
Suite 300
Bethesda, MD 20814-3015
301/854-6549

Association of Birth Defect
Children
3526 Emerywood Lane
Orlando, FL 32812
407/859-2821

ARC
P.O. Box 300649
Arlington, TX 76010
817/261-6003
817/277-0553

Autism Society of America
8601 Georgia Ave.
Suite 503
Silver Spring, MD 20901
301/565-0433

Council for Exceptional
Children
1920 Association Dr.
Reston, VA 22091
703/620-3660

Cystic Fibrosis Foundation
6931 Arlington Rd.
Second Floor
Bethesda, MD 20814-5200
301/951-4422

Epilepsy Foundation of America
4351 Garden City Dr.
Suite 406
Landover, MD 20785
800/332-1000
301/459-3700

ERIC Clearinghouse on
Handicapped and Gifted
Children
Council for Exceptional
Children
1920 Association Dr.
Reston, VA 22091-1539
703/620-3660

Federation for Children with
Special Needs
Suite 104
95 Berkeley St.
Boston, MA 02116
617/482-2915

Gifted Child Society
190 Rock Rd.
Glen Rock, NJ 07452
201/444-6530

Head Start Project
Department of Health and
 Human Services
P.O. Box 1182
Washington, DC 20013
800/245-0572
202/245-0572

International Center for the
 Disabled
340 E. Twenty-fourth St.
New York, NY 10010-4019
212/679-0100

International Rett Syndrome
 Assn.
8511 Rose Marie Dr.
Fort Washington, MD 20744
301/248-7031

Learning Disability Association
 of America
4156 Liberty Rd.
Pittsburgh, PA 15234
412/341-1515
412/341-8077

March of Dimes Foundation
1275 Mamaroneck Ave.
White Plains, NY 10605
914/428-7100

Muscular Dystrophy Association
3561 E. Sunrise Dr.
Tucson, AZ 85718
800/223-6666

National Association for Parents
 of the Visually Impaired
P.O. Box 317
Watertown, MA 02272
800/562-6265

National Association for
 the Deaf
814 Thayer Ave.
Silver Spring, MD 20910
301/587-1788
301/587-1789 (TDY)

National Down Syndrome
 Congress
1800 Dempster St.
Park Ridge, IL 60068-1146
800/232-NDSC
708/823-7550

National Down Syndrome
 Society
666 Broadway
New York, NY 10012
800/221-4602
212/460-9330

National Easter Seal Society
2023 W. Ogden Ave.
Chicago, IL 60612
800/336-4797
312/726-6200

National Health Information
 Center
P.O. Box 1133
Washington, DC 20013-1133
800/336-4797
301/656-4167

National Information Center for
Children and Youth with
Disabilities
P.O. Box 1492
Washington, DC 20013-1492
800/999-5599
703/893-8614 (TDD)

National Information Center
on Deafness*
800 Florida Ave., N.E.
Washington, DC 20002
202/651-5051
202/651-5052 (TDD)

National Library Services for the
Blind and Physically
Handicapped
The Library of Congress
Washington, DC 20542
800/424-8567
800/424-9100 (TDD English)
800/345-8901 (TDD Spanish)
202/707-5100

National Maternal and Child
Health Clearinghouse*
Thirty-eighth and R Sts., N.W.
Washington, DC 20057
202/625-8410

National Rehabilitation
Information Center
8455 Colesville Rd.
Suite 935
Silver Spring, MD 20910-3319
800/346-2742 (TDD)
301/588-9284

Orton Dyslexia Society
Chester Building #382
8600 LaSalle Rd.
Baltimore, MD 21204
800/222-3123
410/296-0232

Special Wish Foundation
2244 S. Hamilton
Columbus, OH
614/575-9474

Sibling Information Network
University of Connecticut
Affiliated Program
991 Main St.
Suite 3A
East Hartford, CT 06108
203/282-7050

Sick Kids (Need) Involved
People
990 Second Ave.
Second Floor
New York, NY 10022
212/421-9160
212/421-9161

Special Olympics
1350 New York Ave.
Suite 500
Washington, DC 20005-4709
202/628-3630

Spina Bifida Association of
  America
4590 MacArthur Blvd., N.W.
Suite 250
Washington, DC 20007
800/621-3141
202/944-3285

Texas Respite Resource Network
512/228-0688

United Cerebral Palsy
  Association
435–437 Maryland Ave.
Essex, MD 21221
410/574-7696

*National Clearinghouses

GLOSSARY

The terms are defined in relation to use in this book and are by no means complete definitions.

Abortion: loss of a pregnancy before viability (twenty-four weeks).

Abruptio placentae: premature separation of the placenta from the uterus.

Aerobic: requiring physical exertion and energy.

Agglutinate: to cause red blood cells to clump together.

Alimentary canal: the digestive system.

Allele: one of two genes, found on a chromosome, that causes specific characteristics, such as eye color.

Alpha-fetoprotein: a substance secreted by the fetus and found in the amniotic fluid and the mother's blood.

Amniocentesis: the removal and examination of a small amount of amniotic fluid to determine genetic and other disorders in the fetus.

Amnion: a thin, tough membranous sac that surrounds the embryo and fetus.

Amniotomy: artificial rupture of membranes.

Analgesic: a medication that relieves or reduces pain.

Androgen: a hormone, such as testosterone, that controls and maintains male characteristics.

Anemia: a decrease in red blood cells, which carry oxygen in the blood.

Anencephaly: an absence of most or all of the brain.

Anesthesia: partial or complete loss of pain, with or without loss of consciousness.

Anterior: the front of the body.

Antibiotic: a medication that kills or reduces the amount of bacteria.

Antibody: protein that forms the basis of immunity. It is produced by the body in response to specific substances, such as bacteria or antigens.

Anticonvulsant: a drug that prevents or relieves convulsions.

Antigen: a substance that stimulates the production of antibodies.

Apgar score: a system of assessing the general physical condition of a newborn.

Arrest of descent: when a fetus stops descending into the vagina.

Artificial insemination: introduction of semen into the vagina or uterus without sexual intercourse.

Atony: lack of muscle tone.

Augmentation: the addition of pitocin to strengthen or increase the number of contractions.

Bacteriostatic: substance that kills bacteria.

Basal body temperature: the temperature obtained upon awakening and before physical activity has begun.

Beta blocker: a drug used for the treatment of hypertension and heart disease.

Bilirubin: a substance produced by the breakdown of red blood cells.

Biopsy: a sample of tissue removed for diagnostic purposes.

Blastocyst: the fertilized egg after a number of cell divisions.

Blighted ovum: a fertilized egg that produces a placenta but no fetus.

Blood pressure: a measurement of the work of the heart and the pressure of blood against the walls of the blood vessels.

Blood type: the specific class of blood based on the presence or absence of antigens on the red blood cells. The main groups are A, B, AB and O.

Braxton-Hicks contractions: irregular, intermittent contractions of the uterus that do not cause dilation and effacement of the cervix.

B-strep: a type of bacteria.

Carpal tunnel syndrome: compression of a nerve going to the hand that results in pain, tingling and numbness of the fingers.

Catheter: a hollow, flexible tube inserted to drain the bladder.

Cephalopelvic disproportion: when the head of the fetus is too large to fit through the mother's pelvis.

Cerclage: stitches placed around the cervix to keep the cervix closed. Used to treat cervical incompetence.

Cervicitis: inflammation of the cervix.

Cervix: the neck-shaped opening of the uterus.

Chlamydia: a sexually transmitted disease.

Chorioamnionitis: an inflammation and infection of the membranes that surround the fetus.

Chorion: the outer membrane surrounding the fetus.

Chorionic villus sapling: a test used to detect birth defects in which a small amount of placental tissue is removed from the uterus.

Chromosome: the structure in the nucleus of a cell that carries hereditary factors.

Cilia: hairlike projections.

Circumcise: removal of the foreskin from the penis.

CMV: cytomegalovirus, a virus that causes birth defects in the fetus if acquired by the mother during pregnancy.

Colic: severe abdominal pain usually caused by gas.

Colostrum: the thin, protein-rich fluid that precedes the production of true milk.

Congenital abnormality: an abnormality present at birth and acquired during uterine development. It can be the result of disease, drugs or an abnormal gene.

Contraction stress test (CST): a test of the fetus's response to contractions.

Convulsion: a seizure.

Cordocentesis: a test that involves obtaining a blood sample from the umbilical cord while the fetus is still in utero.

Corpus luteum: the mass of cells that form from the ovarian follicle after release of an egg that produces progesterone.

Couvade syndrome: a phenomenon in which men show the symptoms of pregnancy.

Crown-rump length: measurement from the top of the head to the bottom of the rump of the fetus.

Crowning: when the head is seen at the opening of the vagina.

Cryosurgery: freezing of the cervix to eliminate abnormal tissue.

Cystic fibrosis: a hereditary disease that affects the lungs.

Cytomegalovirus: see *CMV.*

DES: a synthetic estrogen once used to prevent miscarriages. It is no longer used because it caused structural abnormalities in the sons and daughters of the mothers who took the drug.

Diuretic: a medication used to treat hypertension that reduces the body's fluid volume.

Doppler: a device used to listen to the fetal heartbeat.

Doula: a woman hired as a postpartum mother's helper.

Down's syndrome: a genetic abnormality caused by an extra chromosome 21, which causes mental retardation and other physical abnormalities.

Dysmenorrhea: painful menstruation.

Eclampsia: a severe form of preeclampsia in which coma and convulsions may be present.

Ectopic pregnancy: implantation and development of a fertilized ovum outside the uterus.

Embryo: the name given to the fertilized egg from implantation through the eighth week of pregnancy.

Endometriosis: the presence of endometrial tissue outside the uterus.

Endometrium: the tissue that lines the uterus.

Engagement: the presenting part of the baby as it descends into the pelvis.

Enzyme: a protein substance that acts as a catalyst.

Epidural anesthesia: anesthesia produced by the injection of local anesthetic into the epidural space of the spine.

Epilepsy: a neurological disorder in which seizures occur.

Episiotomy: incision made in the perineum to facilitate delivery.

Essential hypertension: hypertension without apparent cause.

Estrogen: a hormone produced by the ovaries that contributes to the monthly preparation of the uterus for pregnancy and promotes the development and maintenance of female sex characteristics.

Fallopian tubes: the two tubes extending one from each side of the uterus through which an egg travels after release from the ovary. Fertilization usually occurs here.

Fetoscopy: looking at the fetus in utero with a fiber-optic device.

Fetus: an unborn baby after the eighth week of pregnancy.

Fibroid: a noncancerous, ball-shaped growth of muscle fiber that can occur in the uterus.

Fimbria: the fingerlike projections at the end of the fallopian tubes.

Folic acid: a B-complex vitamin that is essential for healthy growth of the fetus.

Fontanelles: the soft spots on the baby's head.

Forceps: tonglike device used to assist in delivery.

Foreskin: the loose tissue that covers the head of the penis.

Formula: a liquid food for babies, containing most of the nutrients found in breast milk.

Fundus: the top of the uterus.

Gestation: pregnancy.

GIFT: gamete intrafallopian transfer.

Glucose: the principal circulating sugar in the blood and the major energy source of the body.

Gonorrhea: a sexually transmitted disease.

Gravity: a term meaning the number of pregnancies a woman has had.

Halothane: an anesthetic gas.

HCG: see *Human chorionic gonadotropin.*

Hematocrit: the volume of red blood cells in the blood.

Hemoglobin: the iron-containing pigment in red blood cells that assists in carrying oxygen throughout the body.

Hemolytic anemia: anemia caused by destruction of red blood cells.

Hemophilia: a hereditary blood coagulation disorder that is manifested almost exclusively in males.

Hemorrhage: excessive loss of blood.

Hemorrhoids: dilated or swollen veins in the anus that can be itchy and painful.

Hepatitis: an inflammation of the liver caused by infection.

Herpes: a viral infection that causes blisters on the skin or mucus membranes.

Hormone: a substance produced by one tissue and conveyed by the blood to another tissue to stimulate activity in that tissue.

Human chorionic gonadotropin (HCG): a substance produced by the placenta that maintains the corpus luteum, causing it to produce progesterone during pregnancy.

Hydronephrosis: enlargement of the kidney due to obstruction of the bladder or ureters.

Hyperemesis gravidarum: excessive vomiting during pregnancy.

Hyperglycemia: excessive, abnormal amounts of glucose in the blood.

Hypertension: high blood pressure.

Hypotension: low blood pressure.

Hypoxemia: insufficient oxygen in the blood.

Implantation: nesting of the fertilized egg into the uterine lining.

Impotent: incapable of sexual intercourse.

Incision: a surgical cut.

Induction: artificial starting of labor.

Infertility: inability to reproduce.

Inherit: to receive a characteristic from one's parents by genetic transmission on the genes of the chromosome.

Insulin: a substance that controls the body's use of glucose.

Intubate: to put a tube in the throat to assist breathing or examine the vocal cords.

In vitro fertilization (IVF): fertilization of the egg outside the body.

Involution of the uterus: a decrease in the size of the uterus to normal size following childbirth.

Ionizing radiation: high-energy radiation that may cause damage to human tissue.

Jaundice: a yellow coloring of the skin and whites of the eyes caused by excess bilirubin in the blood.

Laceration: a tear.

Lactation: formation of milk by the breasts.

Lanugo: a covering of soft, fine hair on the newborn.

Laparoscopy: a surgical procedure in which a slender tube is placed through an incision to examine or perform surgery on tissue inside the abdomen or pelvis.

Linea nigra: a darkened line that appears on the abdomen during pregnancy.

Lithotomy position: a position in which a woman lies on her back with legs held up by assistance.

Lochia: the discharge present after delivery.

Macrosomia: excessive size.

Manic-depressive: a mental disorder characterized by alternating periods of elation and depression.

Meconium: the dark green, sticky bowel contents of the baby at birth.

Meconium aspiration: the breathing of meconium-containing fluid by the baby at birth.

Meditation: the act or process of contemplation.

Menopause: permanent cessation of monthly egg production and menstruation.

Menstruation: the monthly flow of blood from the uterus if pregnancy does not occur.

Metabolism: the process by which the body turns food into fuel for energy.

Miscarriage: see *Abortion.*

Mitral valve prolapse: a condition in which the mitral valve of the heart does not close properly.

Mittelschmerz: the discomfort some women feel at the time ovulation occurs.

Molding: the shaping and compression of the presenting part of the baby as it passes through the vagina during birth.

Morning sickness: nausea and vomiting during pregnancy.

Mucus: a sticky substance that acts as a protective lubricant coating, produced by glands.

Multiple sclerosis: a chronic degenerative disease of the spinal cord and brain.

Myomectomy: removal of fibroids from the uterus.

Neural tube defects (NTD): an abnormality of the spinal cord or brain.

Non-stress test (NST): a test of fetal well-being in which the effect of movement on the heart rate is assessed.

Nonviable: incapable of living.

Occiput: the back part of the head.

Oligohydramnios: abnormally small amount of amniotic fluid.

Ovary: the female reproductive organ that produces the ovum, progesterone and estrogen.

Ovulate: the release of an egg, or ovum, from the ovary.

Ovum: the egg; female gamete.

Oxytocin: a substance produced in the brain that causes contractions of the uterus for labor and signals the breasts to release milk.

Parity: the number of children borne by a woman.

Parturition: the process of giving birth.

Perineum: the area between the vagina and rectum.

Pigmentation: the coloring of the tissues.

Pitocin: a synthetic oxytocin.

Placenta previa: placental tissue covering the opening of the cervix.

Polyhydramnios: excessive amount of amniotic fluid.

Postcoital test: a physical and microscopic examination completed after sexual intercourse.

Posterior: facing or located in the rear of the body.

Postpartum: after delivery.

Preeclampsia: an illness of pregnancy characterized by high blood pressure, swelling or edema, and proteinuria.

Prenatal: existing or occurring during pregnancy.

Progesterone: a hormone produced by the corpus luteum and placenta that prepares the uterus for pregnancy, maintains the pregnancy and promotes development of the breast.

Prostaglandin: hormonelike substance.

Protein: a component of living cells necessary for the proper functioning, growth and repair of tissue.

Proteinuria: the presence of protein in urine.

Puberty: the age of development in which an individual becomes capable of sexual reproduction.

Recto-vaginal fistula: an abnormal connection between the vagina and rectum.

Respirator: a machine that assists breathing.

Respiratory distress syndrome: a respiratory disease of newborns, especially premature babies.

Retinaculum: bandlike structure at the wrist.

RH factor: a substance found on the red blood cells of Rh positive individuals.

Rhogam: a substance that prevents antibodies against Rh factor from forming.

Rubella: a mild, contagious viral rash capable of producing birth defects in babies born to mothers infected during pregnancy. Also called German measles.

Schizophrenia: a mental disorder characterized by withdrawal from reality, illogical patterns of thinking, delusions and hallucinations.

Sedative: a drug that calms and may induce sleep.

Seizure: a convulsion.

Sexually transmitted disease: a disease contracted through sexual intercourse.

Sickle cell disease: a chronic, usually fatal anemia, occurring almost exclusively in blacks of African descent.

Silastic: a silicone material.

Sonogram: an image produced by ultrasound.

Speculum: an instrument inserted into the vagina to view the cervix.

Sphincter: a ring of muscle that controls an opening.

Spider veins: thin veins at the surface of the skin.

Spinal anesthesia: anesthesia injected into the spinal fluid.

Stillbirth: a fetus dead at birth.

Stress: a state of extreme pressure or strain.

Symptom: a sign or indication of a disorder or disease.

Syphilis: a sexually transmitted disease.

Suture: a surgical stitch.

Tay-Sachs disease: a hereditary disease that affects children of Eastern European Jewish parents characterized by mental retardation, convulsions, blindness and, ultimately, death.

Testes: the reproductive organs of the male that produce sperm and testosterone.

Testosterone: hormone produced in the testes responsible for sperm maturation and male sex characteristics.

Thalassemia: an inherited anemia found chiefly among people of Mediterranean descent.

Thrombophlebitis: blood clot in a vein.

Titer: the concentration of a substance in a solution.

Tocolytic: a medication that stops or slows contractions.

Toxemia: see *Preeclampsia.*

Toxoplasmosis: a disease carried in cat feces that can be passed to humans and can cause birth defects in the fetus if the mother contracts the disease during pregnancy.

Transfuse: to give blood or blood products.

Tuberculosis: an infectious disease characterized by coughing, fever, night sweats and weight loss.

Umbilical cord: the cordlike structure connecting the fetus to the placenta.

Urethra: the canal through which urine is passed out of the body.

Uric acid: a breakdown product of protein metabolism.

Urinalysis: test of the urine for bacteria, protein and glucose.

Vascular: containing blood vessels.

Vas deferens: the tube through which semen is carried to the urethra.

Vernix: the waxy, protective coating covering the skin of the fetus.

Vertex: the top of the head.

Yoga: a system of exercises practiced to promote control of the mind and body.

ZIFT: zygote intrafallopian transfer.

BIBLIOGRAPHY

Academic American Encyclopedia, online edition. Danbury, CT: Grolier Electronic Publishing, 1993.

Arrigo, Mary. "MotherCare: Spoiled Milk?" *Parenting* 192 (June/July): 56.

Assennato, G., et al. "Sperm Count Suppression without Endocrine Dysfunction in Lead-Exposed Men." *Archives of Environmental Health* 41(6): 30, 90.

Barr, H. M., and A. P. Streissguth. "Caffeine Use during Pregnancy and Child Outcome: A 7-Year Prospective Study." *Neurotoxicology and Teratology* 13(4): 441–448.

Barrett, Mary Elin. "Medical Ethics: The Hardest Decision a Mother Could Make, Impossible Choices of Prenatal Testing." *McCall's* (March 1992): 44, 46, 48, 50–52, 141.

Barron, William, and Marshall Lindheimer. *Medical Disorders during Pregnancy.* St. Louis: Mosby Year Book, 1991.

Bauman, Andrea. "Second-Hand Stress." *American Health: Fitness of Body and Mind* (April 1991): 74.

Bean, Constance. *Methods of Childbirth,* rev. ed. New York: Quill, William Morrow, 1990.

Berezin, Judith. *The Complete Guide to Child Care.* New York: Random House, 1990.

Blackburn, Susan, and Donna Loper. *Maternal, Fetal, and Neonatal Physiology: A Clinical Perspective.* Philadelphia: W. B. Saunders, 1992.

Bracken, M. B., et al. "Association of Cocaine Use with Sperm Concentration, Motility, and Morphology." *Fertility and Sterility* 53(2): 315–322.

Brent, R. L., and D. A. Beckman. "Environmental Teratogens." *Bulletin of the New York Academy of Medicine* 66(2): 123–163.

Briggs, Gerald, Roger Freeman, and Sumner Yaffe. *Drugs in Pregnancy and Lactation.* Baltimore: Williams & Wilkins, 1990.

Brown, M. A., et al. "Extracellular Fluid Volumes in Pregnancy-Induced Hypertension." *Journal of Hypertension* 10(1): 61–68.

Cherry, Sheldon. "Who Should Deliver Your Baby?" *Parents* (February 1992): 152, 154.

————. "Sex after the Baby." *Parents* (June 1992): 158 (February 1992: 152, 154).

Cordero, J. F. "Effect of Environmental Agents on Pregnancy Outcomes: Disturbances of Prenatal Growth and Development." *Medical Clinics of North America* 74(2): 279–290.

Corner, Anne-Marie. "When You're CEO—and Pregnant." *Working Woman* (September 1992): 39–40.

Coste, J., et al. "Increased Risk of Ectopic Pregnancy with Maternal Cigarette Smoking." *American Journal of Public Health* 81(2): 199–201.

Crane, M. J. "The Diagnosis and Management of Maternal and Congenital Syphilis." *Journal of Nurse Midwifery* 37(1): 4–16.

Cunningham, F. Gary, Paul MacDonald, and Norman Gant. *Williams Obstetrics,* 18th ed. Norwalk, CT: Appleton & Lange, 1989.

Davidoff, Esther. "The Breastfeeding Taboo." *Redbook* (July 1992): 92–95, 114.

Dawes, M. G., and J. G. Grudzinskas. "Patterns of Maternal Weight Gain in Pregnancy." *British Journal of Obstetrics and Gynecology* 98(2): 195–201.

Day, N., et al. "Prenatal Marijuana Use and Neonatal Outcome." *Neurotoxicology and Teratology* 13(3): 329–334.

Deter, R. L., et al. "Neonatal Growth Assessment Score: A New Approach to the Detection of Intrauterine Growth Retardation in the Newborn." *American Journal of Obstetrics and Gynecology* 162(4): 1030–1036.

Dildy, G. A., et al. "Amniotic Fluid Volume Assessment: Comparison of Ultrasonographic Estimates versus Direct Measurements with a Dye-Dilution Technique in Human Pregnancy." *American Journal of Obstetrics and Gynecology* 167(4): 986–994.

Donald, J. M., et al. "Reproductive and Developmental Toxicity of Toluene: A Review." *Environmental Health Perspective* 94: 237–244.

Eden, Alvin. "How to Choose Your Baby's Doctor." *American Baby* (January 1992): 10, 37.

Eiger, Marvin, and Sally Wendkos Olds. "A Man's Role in Breastfeeding." *American Baby* (June 1987): 37, 73–75.

Eriksen, G., et al. "Placental Abruption: A Case-Control Investigation." *British Journal of Obstetrics and Gynecology* 98(5): 448–452.

Eskenazi, B., et al. "A Multivariate Analysis of Risk Factors for Preeclampsia." *JAMA* 266(2): 237–241.

Fancher, Vivian Kramer. *Safe Kids: A Complete Child Safety Handbook and Resource Guide for Parents.* New York: John Wiley and Sons, 1991.

Fingerhut, L. A., et al. "Smoking before, during and after Pregnancy." *American Journal of Public Health* 80(5): 541–544.

Foley, Denise, and Susan Godbey. "Women's Health: Primetime Pregnancy." *Prevention* (October 1992): 52–57, 124–128.

Gabbe, Steven, Jennifer Niebyl, and Joe Leigh Simpson. *Obstetrics: Normal and Problem Pregnancies,* 2nd ed. New York: Churchill Livingstone, 1991.

General Information, Inc., eds. *America's Phone Book.* New York: Simon & Schuster, 1989.

Geschwind, S. A., et al. "Risk of Congenital Malformations Associated with Proximity to Hazardous Waste Sites." *American Journal of Epidemiology* 135(11): 1197–1207.

Granat, Diane. "Precious Lives, Painful Choices." *The Washingtonian* (January 1991): 94–97, 164–171.

Hakim, R. B., and J. M. Tielsch. "Maternal Cigarette Smoking during Pregnancy: A Risk Factor for Childhood Strabismus." *Archives of Ophthalmology* 110(10): 1459–1462.

Hall, Nancy. "A Newborn's First Exam." *American Baby* (April 1992): 82, 84, 120.

Harger, J. H., et al. "Risk Factors for Preterm Rupture of Fetal Membranes: A Multi-center Case Control Study." *American Journal of Obstetrics and Gynecology* 163(1): 130–137.

Harrison, Michael, Mitchell Golbus, and Roy Filly. *The Unborn Patient: Prenatal Diagnosis and Treatment.* Philadelphia: W. B. Saunders, 1991.

Heinonen, O. P., S. Slone, and S. Shapiro. *Birth Defects and Drugs in Pregnancy.* Littleton, MA: Publishing Sciences Group, 1977.

Heins, Henry. "Dear Doctor: Prenatal Blood and Urine Tests." *American Baby* (August 1990): 23–25.

———. "Your Healthy Pregnancy: Late-Pregnancy Tests: Who Needs Them and Why." *American Baby* (July 1992): 22, 24.

Hollingsworth, Dorothy Reycroft. *Pregnancy, Diabetes and Birth,* 2nd ed. Baltimore: Williams & Wilkins, 1992.

Hotchner, Tracy. "Alternative Birth: Have It Your Way." *New West* (January 3, 1977): 55–58.

Institute of Medicine. *Nutrition during Pregnancy and Lactation.* Washington, DC: National Academy Press, 1992.

Jimenez, Sherry. "Breastfeeding: Fact and Fiction." *American Baby* (March 1991): 48, 96, 98–99.

———. "When Your Belly Button Hurts." *American Baby* (February 1992): 46–50, 66.

Joesoef, M. R., et al. "Are Caffeinated Beverages Risk Factors for Delayed Conception?" *Lancet* 335(8682): 136–137.

Karp, Marshall. "66 Things Your Father Never Taught You." *Parents* (June 1992): 107–108, 110.

Keleher, K. C. "Occupational Health: How Work Environments Can Affect Reproductive Capacity and Outcome." *Nurse Practitioner* 16(1): 23–30, 33–34, 37.

Kelly, Margarite, and Elia Parsons. *The Mother's Almanac,* rev. ed. New York: Doubleday, 1992.

Lesko, Matthew. *Lesko's Info Power.* Kensington, MD: Information USA, 1990.

Levine, Michael. *The Address Book.* New York: Perigee Books, 1993.

Lindbohm, M. L., et al. "Magnetic Fields of Video Display Terminals and Spontaneous Abortion." *American Journal of Epidemiology* 136(9): 1041–1051.

Miller, W. H., and M. C. Hyatt. "Perinatal Substance Abuse." *American Journal of Drug and Alcohol Abuse* 18(3): 247–61.

Mittlemark, Raul, Robert Wiswell, and Barbara Drinkwater. *Exercise in Pregnancy.* Baltimore: Williams & Wilkins, 1991.

Moore, Keith. *The Developing Human,* 2nd ed. Philadelphia: W. B. Saunders, 1977.

Nandi, C., and M. R. Nelson. "Maternal Pregravid Weight, Age, and Smoking Status as Risk Factors for Low Birth Weight Births." *Public Health Report* 107(6): 658–662.

Nilsson, Lennart. *A Child Is Born.* New York: Delta/Seymour Lawrence Book, 1990.

O'Connell, C. M., and P. A. Fried. "Prenatal Exposure to Cannabis: A Preliminary Report of Postnatal Consequences in School-age Children." *Neurotoxicology and Teratology* 13(6): 631–639.

Paul, Maureen. *Occupational and Environmental Reproductive Hazards.* Baltimore: Williams & Wilkins, 1993.

Petitti, D. B., and C. Coleman. "Cocaine and the Risk of Low Birthweight." *American Journal of Public Health* 80(1): 25–28.

Price, Anne, and Nancy Dana. "A Guide to Weaning Your Baby." *American Baby* (November 1990): 60, 62.

Roberts, W. E., et al. "The Incidence of Preterm Labor and Specific Risk Factors." *Obstetrics and Gynecology* 76(1 Suppl.): 855–895.

Rosen, M. "Preconception Care: Why It Is Necessary." *The Female Patient* 15(5): 74, 76, 78–79.

Salmon, Dena. "Parents Guide: Breast and Bottle Feeding." *Parents* (September 1992): 141–148.

Schorr, T. M., et al. "Video Display Terminals and the Risk of Spontaneous Abortion." *New England Journal of Medicine* 324(11): 727–733.

Seligmann, Jean, et al. "Is My Baby All Right?" *Newsweek* (June 22, 1992): 62–63.

Shapiro, Jerrold. *When Men Are Pregnant: Needs and Concerns of Expectant Fathers.* San Luis Obispo, CA: Impact Publishers, 1987.

Simpson, Joe Leigh, and Mitchell Golbus. *Genetics in Obstetrics and Gynecology,* 2nd ed. Philadelphia: W. B. Saunders, 1992.

Singer, L., et al. "Childhood Medical and Behavioral Consequences of Maternal Cocaine Use." *Journal of Pediatrics* 17(4): 389–406.

Slutsker, L. "Risks Associated with Cocaine Use during Pregnancy." *Obstetrics and Gynecology* 79(5): 778–789.

Springer, N. S., et al. "Using Early Pregnancy Weight Gain and Other Nutrition-related Risk Factors to Predict Pregnancy Outcomes." *Journal of the American Dieticians Association* 92(2): 217–219.

Stene, J. Fischer, et al. "Paternal Age Effect in Down's Syndrome." *American Journal of Human Genetics* 40: 299.

Stevenson-Smith, Fay, and Dean Salmon. "Is Your Workplace Safe?" *Parents* (September 1992): 219, 225.

Symposium. "Why It's Important to Help Patients Prepare for Pregnancy." *Contemporary OB/GYN* 33(6): 2–14.

Thomas, Clayton L., ed. *Tabor's Cyclopedic Medical Dictionary,* seventeenth ed. Philadelphia: F. A. Davis, 1993.

Vio, F., et al. "Smoking during Pregnancy and Lactation and Its Effects on Breast-milk Volume." *American Journal of Clinical Nutrition* 54(6): 1011–1016.

Vogt, M. J., et al. "Sperm Quality of Healthy Smokers, Ex-Smokers, and Never-Smokers." *Fertility and Sterility* 45(1): 106–110.

Volpe, J. J. "Effect of Cocaine Use on the Fetus." *New England Journal of Medicine* 327(6): 399–407.

Weitzman, M., et al. "Maternal Smoking and Behavior Problems of Children." *Pediatrics* 90(3): 342–349.

Williams, M. A., et al. "Cigarette Smoking during Pregnancy in Relation to Placenta Previa." *American Journal of Obstetrics and Gynecology* 165(1): 28–32.

Winthrop, Anne. "Medical Update." *American Baby* (February 1992): 10.

Winick, Myron. *Nutrition, Pregnancy, and Early Infancy.* Baltimore: Williams & Wilkins, 1989.

Woessner, Candace, Judith Lauwers, and Barbara Bernard. *Breastfeeding Today: A Mother's Companion.* Garden City Park, NY: Avery Publishing Group, 1991.

Yazigi, R. A., et al. "Demonstration of Specific Binding of Cocaine to Human Spermatozoa." *JAMA* 266(14): 1956–1959.

Zimmerman, E. F. "Substance Abuse in Pregnancy: Teratogenesis." *Pediatrics* 20(10): 541–544.

INDEX